# Gene Mapping
in
## Laboratory Mammals

## Part A

# Gene Mapping
# in
# Laboratory Mammals, v. 1

## Part A

by

Roy Robinson

℗ PLENUM PRESS ·London—New York·1971

Plenum Publishing Company Ltd.
Davis House
8 Scrubs Lane
Harlesden
London NW10 6SE
Tel: 01-969 4727

U.S. Edition published by
Plenum Publishing Corporation
227 West 17th Street
New York New York 10011

SBN: 306-37551-6
Library of Congress Catalog Card Number: 73-178776

Printed in Great Britain by
The Whitefriars Press Ltd., London and Tonbridge

# Preface

The present work is an attempt to provide a systematic treatment of genetic linkage in diploid heredity. Part A presents a general account of statistical methods which can be brought to bear on the problem. The primary emphasis is on the practical aspects of estimation. A large proportion, if not the majority, of mutant genes fail to match up to 'textbook' genes—with faultless segregation ratios and expression—yet, these are the materials with which the practical researcher has to cope. For this reason, it is important to know how to deal with the assortment of genes which may display significant deviations from expectation.

Part B examines the accumulated data on linkage for most of the laboratory mammals and provides a comprehensive and up-to-date survey. The need for a critical review has often been expressed and it is hoped that the present analysis will fill the gap. The volume of material is probably the most important in the animal kingdom other than that for *Drosophila* species.

*September, 1971*                                   Roy Robinson

# Acknowledgements

I should like to record my appreciation of the many people who have encouraged and assisted me in the writing of this book. I am indebted to Drs. C. J. Cooksey, D. S. Falconer, P. W. Lane, J. L. Southard and M. E. Wallace for specific acts of assistance. I am obliged to the many investigators who kindly sent me reprints of their published work and, particularly, to those who have generously granted permission to cite unpublished material. I am grateful to Miss M. B. Newcombe for computational assistance.

# Contents of Part A

### Part A: The Biometrical Approach

Contents of Part B: Linkage in Mammalian Species

The following chapter headings will appear in Part B:
House Mouse · Norway Rat · Rabbit · Guinea Pig · Deer-
mouse · Golden Hamster · Cat · Dog · American Mink
Index to Part B · Consolidated Index to Parts A and B.

# Part A

# THE BIOMETRICAL APPROACH

# CHAPTER 1

# Introduction

The concept of linkage was unknown to Gregor Mendel and it must be a moot point whether his analytical mind could have provided the correct explanation for it. As it is, the discovery of associations of genes did in fact open up a temporary false trail (the reduplication hypothesis). However, the realization of the fundamental connection of genes and chromosomes soon led to an appreciation that linkage was the genetic expression of physical change between the chromosome strands. Thus, the final chapter of Mendel's classical exposition of gene assortment was written. Many genes assort independently but, since the number of chromosomes are few and the number of genes per organism are legion, all eventually will fall into definable linkage groups equal in number to the haploid chromosome number.

Most geneticists experience a sense of satisfaction when a mutant gene can be assigned to a linkage group. In principle, this is a simple task. Unfortunately, several factors can intervene. The major one is undoubtedly that of deriving an unbiased estimate of the crossover value. Individual gene ratios can be distorted by inviability, impenetrance, and interactions between these two variables for particular genotypes. The problem is that of allowing for these distortions. In many of the simpler situations this can be achieved without too much trouble, admittedly at the expense of slightly more complex algebraic formulae and sacrifice of statistical information but, usually, this is a small price to pay for reliable estimation.

The emphasis will be on the practical aspects of estimation and special problems which can arise. In general, there will be a progression from the simple to the more complex. Most studies of linkage are two-point but three-point are more valuable, not merely in terms of time and economic deployment of animals, but also by providing information on the strength of interference along the chromosome.

To anticipate the recommendations of the sections which follow, the ideal linkage experiment is (a) a testcross, (b) is appropriately balanced (consisting of equal numbers of coupling and repulsion offspring), and so designed that (c) estimates of the recombination value can be realized for each sex. If the experiment is a three-point cross, the balancing is a little more complex than for a two-point but not onerously so. Also, if a three-point, every endeavour should be made to obtain adequate numbers of the double crossover class so that a meaningful Kosambi coefficient can be calculated. Even if the recombination value between the sexes is not significantly different, the data should not be pooled. The fact of non-significance, especially if the data are extensive enough to reveal anything except a very small difference, could itself be meaningful. Similarly, the values of the Kosambi coefficient should be reported for each sex separately even if these do not differ significantly.

### DEFINITIONS

A number of the terms commonly employed in linkage investigation are sometimes used in different senses by different people. Usually, the differences are subtle rather than a disregard for another person's usage. This sort of semantic variability is probably inevitable to some extent and is certainly not confined to the subject under review (see, for example, the comments of Hollander, 1953, 1955, 1964). However, the arrival of lexicon-cum-encyclopedias of the style of Rieger, Michaelis, and Green (1968) should encourage more uniformity.

The following definitions are used in this work. These follow in many respects the definitions of Carter and Falconer (1952). The backcross to the double recessive is by far the most frequently employed mating in the investigation of linkage. This particular backcross has been termed the testcross and this seems to be an ideal term for linkage work. The word is as simple to use as backcross and preferable to the more cumbersome term double backcross. The latter has been used to distinguish the testcross from the single backcross, in which one gene is backcrossed and the other is intercrossed. The expression single backcross is preferable to mixed cross or single intercross, two alternative terms which have been used for this mating. The expression intercross suffices to define the straight $F_2$ and is preferable to double intercross, an expression which is sometimes used to distinguish the intercross from the single backcross.

There can be three phases of linkage, coupling, repulsion, and mixed, the latter occurring for the special case of the intercross in which one parent is in coupling and the other is in repulsion. It is possible to define coupling in two ways. First, by thinking entirely in terms of mutant genes; whence, both $++/ab$ and $++/A'b$ may be said to be in coupling ($a$, $b$, and $A'$ being mutant genes, the latter a dominant). Or, second, to consider as coupling all those genotypes in which the two dominant genes have been contributed by the same parent, irrespective of which may be the type or mutant. The latter course has been adopted on grounds of consistency. In practice, it has meant that $++/A'b$ must be regarded as in repulsion. The older literature has suffered most from the two interpretations of coupling. Semi-dominant mutant genes should be treated as if they are fully dominant.

The discovery of codominant alleles, such as electrophoretic or immunogenetic variants, for which a 'wild type' is not obvious, raises a problem. One of the alleles will have to be arbitrarily designated as the 'dominant'. The reason is that it may be necessary on occasion to define precisely which alleles have entered a cross from the same parent. This can be stated directly, of course, or it may be convenient to enumerate one cross as 'coupling' and another as 'repulsion' (e.g., for purposes of representation in the abbreviated notation to be discussed anon). It is usual to designate codominant alleles by numerical or lower case Roman letters and it may be proposed that the lower number or earliest letter in the alphabet be regularly chosen as 'dominant'.

Genes which have been derived from the same parent are conventionally separated by an oblique in writing the genotype: $++/ab$ or $a+/+b$, as the case may be. If the genes are linked, this would signify that the genes on either side of the oblique are on the same chromosome. An alternative symbolism is

$$\frac{++}{ab} \quad \text{or} \quad \frac{a+}{+b},$$

employed particularly where genes are definitely known to be linked. This symbolism is useful for tabular presentation but less so for textual.

The abbreviations BC and $F_2$ for the backcross to the recessive parent and for the second filial generation are sufficient for ordinary purposes with assortment of a single gene. However, in linkage analysis, at least two loci are involved. There is also the matter of phase and it is convenient to have a notation which can take these factors into account simultaneously. Phase is commonly denoted by C for coupling and R for repulsion. To these may be added M for the mixed phased intercross. If, now, the backcross is denoted by B and intercross by I with respect to the individual loci in order of writing, the range of possible crosses can be represented as:

CBB   Coupling, both loci backcrossed.
RBB   Repulsion, both loci backcrossed.
CIB   Coupling, first locus intercrossed, second locus backcrossed.
RIB   Repulsion, first locus intercrossed, second locus intercrossed.
CBI   Coupling, first locus backcrossed, second locus intercrossed.
RBI   Repulsion, first locus backcrossed, second locus intercrossed.
CII   Coupling, both loci intercrossed.
RII   Repulsion, both loci intercrossed.
MII   Mixed phase, both loci intercrossed.

Where the sex of the parent contributing crossover gametes can be distinguished, the symbols ♂ and ♀ can be prefixed to the above. Note that the B and I notation can be readily extended for multi-point crosses. The representation of phase for this type of cross is more difficult to denote succinctly. It is recommendable that multi-point crosses should be multiple testcrosses as far as possible. In which case, the respective genes will usually all be in coupling and may be denoted, for example, by ♂CBBB for a male triheterogygous testcross.

The procedures for evaluating the amount of recombination will be described. In every case, a model is proposed from which a parameter, the recombination fraction, will be estimated. To clear the text of unwanted zeros, it is convenient to multiply the fraction by 100. This quantity will be defined as the recombination value. Calculation of the recombination value need not denote linkage. Acceptance of linkage will depend upon the statistical significance of the recombination value and other relevant factors. Once linkage is established, the recombination fraction or value will be spoken of as the crossover fraction or value, respectively.

It is convenient to define two sorts of linkage maps. The first is built up from crossover values, such as the top edge of the trigons featured in later chapters, and the second is a depiction of the loci on the physical chromosome. The first representation could be termed the crossover map since the unit of measure is effectively one crossover unit taken as a percentage. Crossover maps are useful in that they rest entirely upon observation. They suffer, however, a major disadvantage. The intervals between loci are not strictly additive and this often means that the map length will need extension for each new locus.

The second representation is an attempt to avoid this disadvantage by transforming the crossover value into linkage values which are additive. The unit of measure is also a percentage and is the centimorgan (cM). The validity of this type of linkage map rests heavily upon the discovery of a valid transmuting formula or mapping function. Given an accurate function, the resultant map will need either no or only minor revision for each new locus. The transformed map may be termed the chromosome map, care being taken to indicate which mapping function has been employed. No chromosome maps have been drawn up in this survey since it is not clear that a universally acceptable mapping function has been defined. For low crossover values between adjacent loci, the two maps will agree closely.

## GENE EXPRESSION

An attempt is made to introduce a mild degree of order in the mode of expression of the various mutants. The time has passed when the mutant description was a reliable indication of the effect produced. This is still true in large measure, for it is obvious that most workers are at pains to label their mutants descriptively. The other side of the coin is the sheer number of mutants which are known (especially, in the house mouse). This tends to produce a daunting list, particularly for the uninitiated. Partly out of respect for these people and partly because it seems desirable to have some sort of summary classification, the mode of expression of each mutant is noted generally under the heading of prime characteristic in the tables of gene/loci and their symbols.

This classification is certainly not intended to be final although some thinking along these lines would not be out of order. In some respects, the present classification is a little more detailed than other attempts hitherto. Despite this, several broad categories remain, e.g., coat colour and behaviour. The classification is practicable, rather than fundamental, for obvious reasons. Most genes fall naturally into one category but a large number could easily fit into more than one. No real endeavour is made to cope with these. The majority of categories are exclusive but not necessarily. For instance, skeleton could embrace modification of the feet and tail, and hair texture and hypotrichosis could grade into one another. A few mutants could be truly described as physiological but, in practice, this category has tended to be a repository of genes which do not clearly belong to others.

If a summary classification does in fact serve a useful purpose, it seems probable that a comprehensive series of categories will be eventually drafted and most mutants will be ascribed to one (or perhaps to more than one, in exceptional cases), preferably by the discoverer. It was found convenient to adopt the following categories:

| | |
|---|---|
| Coat colour | Body size/growth |
| White spotting | Eye |
| Hair texture | Ear |
| Hypotrichosis | Behaviour |

Skeleton                    Blood
Feet                        Immunogenetics
Tail                        Electrophoretic variants
            Physiology

## LINKAGE TESTING STOCKS

In the past, the majority of linkage studies have been largely opportunist and unplanned. If this charge seems harsh, it must be recognized that this is not always the fault of the experimenter since his primary interest may lie elsewhere. Too often, however, linkage studies with a new mutant have been completed with those other genes which happened to be readily available. Fortunately, the more rational view is gaining ground that the investigation of linkage should be placed on a more systematic basis.

It is easy to be indulgent of past research but a surprising amount of modern work is apt to follow the old pattern. The most elementary requirements of a well conducted linkage experiment are often not fully met. In general, these are two: phase balance and the detection of a sex difference of crossover frequency. For two pairs of genes, phase balance entails setting up of crosses so that equal numbers of progeny are recorded for the two linkage phases. This action tends to minimize inviability effects and interaction between the genes. It is patent that two crosses will suffice in the present instance but the number increases for several pairs of genes if phase balance is to be fully achieved for all genes. See Table 9.1 and associated text for details. Also, the crosses should be so arranged that should linkage be demonstrated, separate estimates of the crossover value can be obtained for each sex.

The logical course is to create stocks of animals containing as many genes as possible which do not interfere with each other in crosses (such as epistatic and inviability interactions). This idea is not new and brief details of four stocks have been given by Cooper (1939) for the mouse. With these stocks, a new mutant could be tested rapidly with 14 other genes; each cross testing three or four genes simultaneously. Further stocks have probably been devised but have not been publicized. However, the problem is complex. For instance, it is obvious that not all mutant genes are suitable for linkage testing. All new mutants, however inviable or epistatic, have to be tested but once the genes have been allocated to a group, some will be seen to be more useful than others.

The theory of the construction of linkage testing stocks has been developed by Carter and Falconer (1951). The number of factors to be considered are basically four. The choice of gene to represent a particular linkage group or segment of chromosome, the type of mating to be employed (e.g., testcross or intercross), the mean number of offspring which can be examined, and the minimum number of stocks which can be formed to yield the maximum amount of information. Most of these variables are interconnected by the concept of the swept radius.

The swept radius is defined as the length of chromosome on either side of a marker gene within which a new mutant can be experimentally excluded. In any test, the null hypothesis is that the two genes are independent or $p = 0.5$. A number of tests would be expected to give values of $p$ distributed around 0.5 by less than $ks$, where $k$ is a constant representing a given level of significance and $s$ is the standard error. Ignoring the possibility of $p$ being greater than 0.5, the limit of swept radius in terms of crossover units is $p_r = 0.05 - ks$. To relate this quantity to chromosome length, it is necessary to adopt a mapping function. For mathematical convenience, Kosambi's function has been chosen.

Therefore, since:

$$x = \frac{1}{4} \ln \frac{1+2p}{1-2p}$$

and substituting:

$$x_r = \frac{1}{4} \ln\left(\frac{\sqrt{I}}{k} - 1\right),$$

where $x_r$ = the limit to the swept radius and $I$ is the amount of information for $p(I = 1/s^2)$. Providing the marker gene does not lie so near the end of the chromosome that the swept radius extends beyond it, the swept distance will be $x_s = 2x_r$ since the new mutant could lie on either side of the marker. The value of

*I* will depend upon the type of mating and upon *n*, the number of offspring examined.

Taking the level of significance at the conventional 5 per cent, $k = 1.65$ for a one-tailed test. The most common linkage test is the testcross, for which $I = in = 4n$. Inserting these quantities in the formulae for the swept distance gives the following for the testcross:

$$x_s = \tfrac{1}{2} \ln\left(\frac{2\sqrt{n}}{1.65} - 1\right).$$

If 70 offspring are examined, corresponding to the detection of linkage of less than 40 per cent, the swept distance is about 110.5 cM of the chromosome. If larger numbers of offspring are examined, the swept distance will obviously be greater. Should other matings be used, $i(=I/n)$ will vary accordingly and should the aim be to detect linkage up to a certain strength, *n* would have to be adjusted to ensure that *I* attains the appropriate level.

The swept distance can be used to resolve several problems which can arise in linkage testing or the development of linkage testing stocks. These involve the choice of alternative marker genes of a linkage group for various situations. Carter and Falconer have considered four general situations and have indicated how a decision can be made. In each case, the deciding factor is the closeness of the loci on the chromosome. This is perhaps obvious but reasonably precise numerical values can be derived. In summary, if two genes are sited on the same chromosome beyond a specified distance, it would be an advantage to incorporate each into the stocks; otherwise the swept distances for each would overlap. Depending on the situation, the distances vary from 10 to 20 cM. The original paper should be consulted for further details.

Carter and Falconer have discussed the formation of linkage testing stocks and the choice of suitable markers from the genes available in the mouse at that time. Eventually, 21 loci were selected and these were allocated to five stocks. Some four to six genes could be tested for linkage with each cross. The chosen genes represented 11 linkage groups and five 'independent' loci, although some of the latter have subsequently been found not to be independent. Subject to certain assumptions, the swept distance for each gene or group of linked genes can be summed to yield a total swept length for the linkage stocks. The total genetic map length of the genome can be conjectured from the mean chiasma frequencies.

The efficiency of a set of stocks could then be assessed by representing the total swept length as a proportion of the total map length. Carter and Falconer found that their proposed stocks are capable of testing a new mutant against about 50 per cent of the genome at the cost of raising a total of 500 offspring. This sort of calculation reveals the power of linkage testing stocks over the orthodox but haphazard methods of linkage detection. Green (1963) has given details of a modern set of seven mouse stocks. These contain 26 loci, representing 16 linkage groups, and the testing efficiency is about 70 per cent of the genome at the cost of examining 700 offspring.

In the construction of the testing stocks, genes with marked inviability of impenetrant effects are clearly unsuitable if better alternatives exist. It is also desirable that phenotypic interaction which can interfere with straightforward classification should be avoided and this aspect, together with the task of combining the genes, will no doubt determine the actual number of stocks. Usually, there is a limit to the number of mutant genes which can be carried by a single stock. Dominant or codominant genes would appear to have definite advantages over recessive and it is doubly advantageous if these are combined in the same stock(s). The reason for this is that different breeding procedures will be demanded depending upon whether the new mutant is dominant or recessive. If the former, testcrosses can be conducted without any difficulty. If the latter, on the other hand, testcrosses can be performed for dominant markers but intercrosses are necessary for recessive. Separation of dominant and recessive markers would mean that no intercrosses need be performed where testcrosses are superior.

As knowledge of the linkage groups expands, existing testing stocks would seemingly become steadily obsolete and new, more efficient, stocks would have to be built up. Ideally, all of the known linkage groups of a species should have at least one representative (depending upon its length), and such other 'independent' genes which may usefully be included. The house mouse has featured prominently in the above discussion but this is because the species is in the forefront of mammalian chromosome mapping. The large number of genes available in the mouse enables very extensive linkage testing stocks to be created but the principle applies equally to a species with few linkage groups but a number of incompletely tested genes waiting to be placed.

It may be mentioned that linkage testing stocks may not be necessarily fully efficient for precise location of a new gene. Their function is primarily that of rapid detection but, once a gene has been shown to be included in a linkage group, further experiments can be set in motion to pin-point the position. In fact, looking ahead, it is possible to perceive the need for a second set of stocks in which groups of linked genes are held available for precise location of new mutants. Three and higher point crosses could be arranged with the objectives of not only locating a new gene but also of gathering information on interference.

## EFFICIENCY OF TESTS

The amount of information contributed by a sample has been defined as the reciprocal of the variance. In fact, the information pertaining to an estimated parameter occurs naturally as part of the maximum likelihood analysis. The amount of information per individual will vary according to the nature of the mating. This has led to the concept of the efficiency of testing. That is, some matings regularly have a smaller variance than others and, by definition, contribute more information per sample. In practice, this means that a smaller sample is required to detect a linkage, to disprove a given linkage value, or to test the significance of a difference.

The efficiency is a relative measure and is conventionally expressed in terms of the mating which would contribute the maximum amount of information. The cross which does this is the fully classified intercross. This is not the same as the intercross with two pairs of codominant genes. Such a cross produces a range of nine different phenotypes but fails to distinguish between the coupling or repulsion phase dihetero-zygote $+a+b$. These have to be distinguished by progeny tests.

The ordinary intercross with two pairs of codominant genes (no progeny testing) actually ranks second.

The testcross ranks third in terms of efficiency. This is interesting on several accounts. Comparison of the efficiency of the fully classified intercross and the testcross reveals that the former is twice as great as the latter over the whole range of

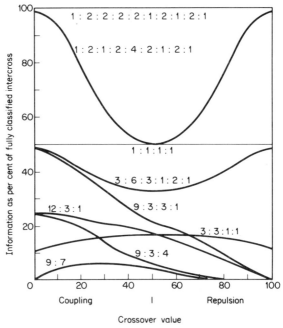

Fig. 1.1 Relative efficiency of various matings in the estimation of the crossover value.

crossover values. No other cross has this property. In other words, either of these matings would be employed as standard. With other crosses, the efficiency varies with the crossover value as shown by Fig. 1.1. It can be seen that the ordinary intercross (no progeny testing) with two pairs of codominant genes is everywhere superior to the testcross, although less so for weak linkage. The peculiar behavior of the curve for the intercross with two dominant genes should be particularly noted. This cross compares favourably with the testcross only for close linkage in coupling. Thereafter, the efficiency falls steadily, being especially poor for close linkage in repulsion. This is another way of saying that the variance has become large and estimates of the crossover value in this region are unreliable.

The relative efficiency of different crosses has been examined by Mather (1936a) but the most comprehensive comparisons are those of Allard (1956). Figure 1.1 summarizes the results for the more important crosses. The omitted curves in the main are those for matings involving epistatic and complementary genes. In general, these crosses have low efficiency over the whole range of crossover values. When these genes have to be investigated, large samples must be examined to yield comparable results.

The effects of inviability and impenetrance on the efficiency have not been investigated in detail. These factors do modify the amount of information but it is improbable that novel effects are introduced. However, it may be thought that an investigation is in order to check the possibility. This is the sort of study which could be most expeditiously handled by a computer programme. The result would be a surface diagram demonstrating the simultaneous variation of the inviability or impenetrance and range of crossover values.

## SEX DIFFERENCES IN CROSSINGOVER

Counts of chiasma frequency between the sexes has provided evidence for a difference of crossingover. The evidence is of general nature, consisting of mean frequencies mostly drawn from bivalents which presented clear configuration. Among the mammals, the mouse and rat have provided the most extensive data. These indicate consistently that the female has a higher chiasma frequency per bivalent and may be expected to have a higher rate of crossingover per intercept on the average. The nature of the observations are such, however, that it would be possible for certain regions of a chromosome, or even certain chromosomes, to behave differently from the average.

The chiasma observations for the mouse have been subjected to an interesting theoretical analysis by Carter (1954). The original paper should be read for exact details but the main features may be noted. The bivalents must be identical for each sex, thus the difference in mean chiasma frequency implies a difference in the interference interval. This means that the chiasma density intervals along the bivalent will vary between the sexes and a high density in one could coincide with a low density in the other. A reversal of the usually higher frequency of crossingover in the female may thus occur. On the data available, Carter's analysis is suggestive that a typical acrocentric chromosome would show a higher rate of crossingover for the female except for a region some 30-50 crossover units from the centromere. The greatest difference of crossingover (in favour of the female) would occur within a short distance from the centromere. Carter's analysis would seem to be quite general. The figures which he derives may need revision in the light of further mouse data or for data from other species.

The importance of Carter's conclusions is that all data on crossingover between the sexes are of value. Since a higher rate of crossingover in the female is almost certainly the rule, exceptions deserve to be noted. Data which show no difference of crossingover between the sexes may, of course, be due to small sample size but these may be indicative of the two points which border the short region of greater crossingover in the male. Information on crossingover between the sexes should be collected as a matter of policy and published in full. A non-significant difference may turn out to be of importance *per se* or attain significance when combined with other data.

Investigation of the influence of sex on the crossover fraction is most easily accomplished by the testcross, employing diheterozygotes of each sex. If this cannot be undertaken because of lethality, sterility, or greatly impaired reproductive ability of one sex, the single backcross can be used. This mating is not so efficient but, at least, the sex difference can be examined.

In principle, the intercross could yield information on the sex difference, provided both coupling and repulsion data are available. However, the numbers required to detect a suspected difference are likely to be considerable. So inordinately large indeed that the method borders on the impractical (Fisher, 1962). However, Fisher makes the point that this disadvantage can be avoided to some extent if sexually reciprocated mixed phase intercrosses can be produced. Large samples would still be required but not of the same magnitude as necessitated by ordinary coupling and repulsion phase samples. The method may be of greater intrinsic interest than of practical application.

In principle, two forms of complete sex-linkage are possible. A group of loci borne by the $X$ chromosome and a group borne by the $Y$. There is also the possibility of partial sex-linkage. No definite instances of the latter mode of heredity have been detected to date. Despite this, the possibility remains. If true homology in the form of a pairing segment exists for the $X$ and $Y$ with exchanges of material and, if the segment contains mutable gene loci, it would seem merely a matter of time before partial sex-linkage is discovered.

$X$ chromosome sex-linkage may be regarded as firmly established. This mode of heredity has been known in the cat (sex-linked orange) since the early days of genetics and in the dog (sex-linked haemophilia) for some three decades. However, there are isolated events and it has fallen to fairly recent research on the mouse to demonstrate that the $X$ differential segment is capable of carrying loci with a variety of functions and that crossingover within it is of regular occurrence. A crossover map comparable to the autosomal linkage group can be built up. Three $X$ borne mutants have since been reported for the golden hamster. It is reasonable to assume, therefore, that similar groups will exist for all or most other mammals. In the mouse, the $X$ linkage group has been designated as the last group (the XXth), perhaps as a mnemonic, and it is recommended that this policy be followed for other species.

$Y$ chromosome linkage must be held to be quite probable but perhaps not more strongly than this at the present time. The only examples of this form of heredity are to be found in the mouse and are possibly not so clearly established as might be desired. The $Y$ chromosome is a variable body, certainly between species and occasionally within species. Only further observations will disclose if the $Y$ differential segment has few or many mutable loci. It would seem that crossingover within the segment is ordinarily impossible and no linkage group can be built up by conventional means.

ZERO CROSSOVERS AND CONFIDENCE LIMITS FOR THE LOW
CROSSOVER VALVES

The problem of the non-recovery of the crossover class for the
repulsion intercross with recessive genes will be discussed in a
succeeding chapter. In essence, this is a special situation since
this particular cross is of poor efficiency. Crossover gametes
may be produced but are obscured by the presence of dominant
alleles. The problem can be handled by a direct test of this
possibility. However, an absence of crossingover may occur for
other situations and it may be wondered if this data can be put
to good use.

It is obvious that no estimate of the crossover function can
be obtained but Stevens (1942) has shown how an idea of the
upper limit can be derived. For the upper limit to have meaning,
the sample must be large and unaffected by an inviability which
could be the primary factor for the absence of the crossover
classes. Stevens provides a table which enables the upper limit
to be found for various probability levels on the assumption of
a Poisson distribution; an extended table is given by Fisher and
Yates (1953). Taking the 5 per cent (two-tailed) as the
traditional significance point and $n$ as the number in sample, the
upper limit $(U)$ in terms of expected number of crossover
individuals is given by:

$$U = 3.69 - \frac{0.64}{n}.$$

The upper limit to the crossover fraction is derived from $U$
but will depend upon the nature of the cross. The testcross
provides the most direct estimate since the expectation for the
sum of the two crossover classes is $np$, hence

$$p = \frac{U}{n}.$$

For the repulsion intercross, the last class will be absent and
the expectation for this will be $np^2/4$, hence:

$$p = \sqrt{\frac{4U}{n}}.$$

In the case of the coupling intercross, the two middle classes will be absent and their expectation is $2np(1-p)$, hence:

$$p = 1 - \sqrt{\left(1 - \frac{2U}{n}\right)}.$$

The double recessive class will be absent in the mixed phase intercross and the expectation is $np(1-p)/4$, hence

$$p = \frac{1 - \sqrt{(1 - 4U/n)}}{2}.$$

The single backcross has only one class which would be lacking as a consequence of a low crossover value. The particular class affected will vary according to the type of single backcross but the expectation, $np$, is identical in each case; hence:

$$p = \frac{U}{n}.$$

The same principle will apply should epistatis be present, provided one class has zero expectancy due to a low rate of crossingover.

The tables prepared by Stevens and by Fisher and Yates may be pressed into service for a related problem. For low crossover values, the usual practice of calculating confidence limits by taking a simple plus and minus multiple of the standard error could be very inaccurate. The distribution of errors is not that of a normal curve but partakes of a skewed binomial or Poisson. A good approximation to the real limits is easily found for the testcross by the method described by Stevens. For a given level of significance, the table is entered for the observed number of crossover individuals. The values for the upper and lower limits set by the table are then divided by the total number of observations to yield the desired limits. If the crossover value is very low, it may be taken as effectively zero with but small error. For larger values, or for more precise calculation, the entries of the table may be interpolated.

## THE PRODUCT FORMULA

An estimating formula which has aroused interest is that known as the product ratio. The interest centres around two aspects of the method. For intercross data, Fisher and Balmukand (1928) showed that the product ratio had the same variance as the maximum likelihood estimator and was, therefore, fully efficient. It was considered that the formula was least affected by possible differential viability (Immer, 1930). The method has been extended to many other matings, particularly by Alam (1929) and Immer (1930). Seal (1957) has discussed an extension of this form of estimation. The efficiency of many of these formulae have not been examined, and may not in fact be very great. Immer (1931) makes the point that the product formula fails when one of the crossover classes equals zero.

The estimating formula for the product ratio is not simpler than the maximum likelihood expression and offers no advantage in calculation. However, its popularity has been boosted by the provision of facilitating tables (Fisher and Balmukand, 1928; Immer, 1930; Stevens, 1939; Immer and Henderson, 1943). All are easy to use and Stevens' is the most comprehensive. The variance for a given $p$ can also be obtained from prepared tables.

The vaunted efficiency of the product ratio may have been overdone. It is as efficient as maximum likelihood estimation for normal intercross gene ratios but less so than the corresponding maximum likelihood expression when allowance is made for inviability of one gene (Fisher, 1939; Bailey, 1949a). When explicit allowance is made for inviability of both genes, the application of maximum likelihood results in a formula identical to the product ratio (but with a complicated expression for the variance). The variance for the product ratio would presumably be the same as that for the maximum likelihood. It is interesting that when due allowance is made for inviability, the two methods assume the same formula. This aspect provides grounds for the belief that the product ratio is less affected by inviability but shows that the product method is not superior to maximum likelihood estimation when inviability is taken fully into account.

## AFFINITY

It is not unknown for certain genes to display quasi-linkage associations despite evidence which is opposed to the possibility that the genes reside in the same chromosomes. This phenomenon, or at least one aspect of it, has been termed affinity. One eminent explanation of quasi-linkage is that certain centromeres are either mutually attracted and tend to travel to the same pole of the cell (mutual affinity) or share a common attraction to some polar element (polar affinity). The first possibility seems to be the more feasible. Genes sited close enough to the centromere to show linkage with it would manifest quasi-linkage. This is the substance of the theory.

Quasi-linkage has been observed in several organisms, notably *Saccharomyces, Drosophila melanogaster*, and the house mouse. The latter species comes within the scope of this book and, without prejudice to work on the phenomenon in other organisms, will be preferentially considered. Michie (1953) and Wallace (1953) have specifically described quasi-linkage in the mouse as affinity. A fuller account will be found in the section on the species. Affinity appears to differ from true linkage in one major respect. There may be association, where the genes tend to stay together (thus mimicking linkage), or there may be dis-association, where the genes tend to repel each other. The latter effect is not readily explicable in terms of true linkage (not always even if crossingover in excess of 50 per cent is accepted) but it would be true in terms of affinity. In essence, association or dis-association denotes the phase of the genes in relation to the centromeres.

The concept of affinity has been developed in detail by Michie (1955), Wallace (1957b, 1958, 1959, 1961), Shult *et al.* (1962, 1967), and Douglas and Geerts (1967). The development of statistical methods for estimation of the amount of crossingover between gene loci and the centromere and the attraction between centromeres from affinity data has been considered by Wallace (1958, 1959, 1961), and Bailey (1961). Two points emerge from these studies. These are (a) the analysis of affinity requires more careful forethought in the design of experiments than the ordinary linkage investigation and (b), unless the experimental design is appropriate, it is often impossible to separate the linkage between gene and centromere from the attraction between centromeres.

The depiction of attraction between the centromeres as the basis of affinity is certainly conceptually satisfying but this assumption is not obligatory. Any site of attraction between chromosomes would foot the bill provided it is constant enough to persist throughout successive investigations. Indeed, independent experiments with translocations in the house mouse have provided evidence for the location of several centromeres which are not in agreement with the position indicated by affinity. This work is still proceeding but it seems probable that the affinity hypothesis in terms of centromeric attraction will have to be modified. It remains to be seen if affinity is due to one or more points of mutual attraction between chromosomes or if a more elaborate theory will have to be formulated.

The expression of affinity thus far has been to simulate either weak linkage or weak super-recombination. The latter, of course, affords a means of distinguishing affinity from linkage. The tendency for weak expression, if it is persistent, is itself a means of identification. In any event, it implies that the observation of weak linkage between a pair of genes is not to be accepted uncritically as evidence of linkage. When affinity is combined with linkage, the effect would be to produce between phase heterogeneity of the crossover values. The detection of the heterogeneity will depend upon the relative magnitudes of the affinity and linkage.

The hypothesis that the centromere is the source of the affinity effect has the merit of being specific. As such, it could expose the hypothesis to more than one experimental attack. For example, the discovery of more than one site of affinity per chromosome would raise grave doubts upon the validity of the centromere concept. Likewise, if a viable acentric chromosome was to display affinity, the possibility of other sites of attraction would have to be taken seriously. It would follow that while the finding of more than one affinity site would not itself disprove that the centromere is involved, it would considerably weaken the idea that the position of the centromere could be derived from an affinity analysis.

CHAPTER 2

# Maximum Likelihood Estimation

It is possible to develop a number of systems of estimation and nowhere does this seem to be more true than for the estimation of genetic crossover fractions. Several of these fail dismally because of inaccuracy and inefficiency (Fisher and Balmukand, 1928). Others have received consideration in the main because of their interesting and special features. These exceptional systems are known as minimum $\chi^2$, product ratio, and minimum discrepancy (Fisher and Balmukand, 1928; Immer, 1930; Haldance,1953; Murty, 1954b). The most versatile and efficient system, however, is the method of maximum likelihood (Fisher, 1922; Mather, 1951; Bailey, 1961). The main objection to the method, namely, that the estimating formulae are often of high degree polynomials, is only correct for a few cases and in the event can be side-stepped by the use of scores.

The method of maximum likelihood consists of the precise description of a sample in terms of the pertinent parameters. For estimation of linkage this means primarily the crossover fraction $(p)$, and the inviability $(v)$ and impenetrance $(\alpha)$, in so far as these are pertinent. The sample will consist of phenotypic classes $m_1 \ldots m_t$ over $t$ classes. This notation will represent the expectations in terms of $p$ ($v$ and $\alpha$ as necessary), summing to unity. The observed frequencies will be denoted as $a, b, \ldots t$ over the same classes, summing to $n$, the number in sample.

## SINGLE PARAMETER

For a given sample, the probability of obtaining a sample of $a$ of the $m_1$ class, . . . and $t$ of the $m_t$ class will be the relevant term of the multinomial expansion:

$$(m_1 + \ldots m_t)^n.$$

The relevant terms is:

$$\frac{n!}{a! \ldots t!} (m_1)^a \ldots (m_t)^t.$$

The method of estimation depends upon the maximization of this term in terms of $p$. In this form, however, the finding of the maximum by differentiation is not easy and it is convenient to transform the term to logarithms before differentiation. The term is rewritten:

$$L = a \ln m_1 + \ldots + t \ln m_t + C,$$

where $C$ represents the factorial component of the term. Differentiating $L$ with respect to $p$ and equating to zero will derive the equation:

$$\frac{dL}{dp} = a \frac{d \ln m_1}{dp} + \ldots + t \frac{d \ln m_t}{dp} = 0.$$

Solving this equation for $p$ will give the value of $p$ which maximizes both $L$ and the multinomial term. This is the required estimating formula for $p$. Since $C$ does not contain $m$ (hence, neither $p$), it vanishes upon differentiation.

The above equation may be written in a more convenient form for algebraic manipulation:

$$\frac{dL}{dp} = \frac{a}{m_1} \frac{dm_1}{dp} + \ldots + \frac{t}{m_t} \frac{dm_t}{dp} = 0.$$

Since the summation is always over the same classes for a sample, the subscripts may be dropped and the above shown as:

$$\frac{dL}{dp} = \Sigma \left( \frac{a}{m} \frac{dm}{dp} \right) = 0.$$

The large sample variance ($V$) of $p$ is not found directly but is derived as its reciprocal. This quantity is known as the amount of information ($I$) relevant to $p$. The inverse relationship between $V$ and $I$ means that the smaller the variance, the greater the amount of information. $I$ represents the total amount of information contributed by the sample. Dividing by the number of observations yields the amount of information ($i$) per single observation ($I/n = i$). The information is defined as the rate of change of $p$ at its maximum value:

$$i = \sum \left( m \frac{\mathrm{d}^2 \ln m}{\mathrm{d}p^2} \right) = \sum \left[ \frac{1}{m} \left( \frac{\mathrm{d}m}{\mathrm{d}p} \right)^2 \right]$$

The estimation proceeds by application of the above formulae. This consists largely of the manipulation of the first derivative of the class expectations. These are usually simple functions of $p$ and such other parameters which are necessary fully to specify the sample. Table 2.1 illustrates the algebra for the analysis of the testcross with normal gene ratios. The expectations are formulated as shown by column $m$ and differentiated to give column $\mathrm{d}m/\mathrm{d}p$. These columns must sum to unity and zero, respectively, and this provides a check on the working. The next column is found by dividing the second into the third. The estimating formula is derived from this column as

TABLE 2.1

Maximum likelihood analysis of the coupling testcross
with normal gene ratios

| Phenotype class | $m$ | $\dfrac{\mathrm{d}m}{\mathrm{d}p}$ | $\dfrac{1}{m}\dfrac{\mathrm{d}m}{\mathrm{d}p}$ | $\dfrac{1}{m}\left(\dfrac{\mathrm{d}m}{\mathrm{d}p}\right)^2$ |
|---|---|---|---|---|
| $++$ | $\dfrac{1-p}{2}$ | $-\dfrac{1}{2}$ | $-\dfrac{1}{1-p}$ | $\dfrac{1}{2(1-p)}$ |
| $+b$ | $\dfrac{p}{2}$ | $\dfrac{1}{2}$ | $\dfrac{1}{p}$ | $\dfrac{1}{2p}$ |
| $a+$ | $\dfrac{p}{2}$ | $\dfrac{1}{2}$ | $\dfrac{1}{p}$ | $\dfrac{1}{2p}$ |
| $ab$ | $\dfrac{1-p}{2}$ | $-\dfrac{1}{2}$ | $-\dfrac{1}{1-p}$ | $\dfrac{1}{2(1-p)}$ |
| Totals | $1$ | $0$ | $-$ | $\dfrac{1}{p(1-p)}$ |

follows: Each term is multiplied by the corresponding observed frequency, summed with due regard to sign, and equated to zero. These operations result in the following:

$$-\frac{a}{1-p}+\frac{b}{p}+\frac{c}{p}-\frac{d}{1-p}=0,$$

whence:

$$p=\frac{b+c}{n}.$$

The variance is found from the fifth column of the table. This is produced by multiplying column four by column three, class by class. The results are summed, as shown by the table. The total gives the amount of information per single observation. This is converted to the total amount of information by multiplying by $n$ and inverted to give:

$$V=\frac{p(1-p)}{n}.$$

TABLE 2.2

Maximum likelihood analysis of the intercross with normal gene ratios

| Class | $m$ | $\dfrac{dm}{dp}$ | $\dfrac{1}{m}\dfrac{dm}{dp}$ | $\dfrac{1}{m}\left(\dfrac{dm}{dp}\right)^2$ |
|---|---|---|---|---|
| $++$ | $\dfrac{2+P}{4}$ | $\dfrac{1}{4}$ | $\dfrac{1}{2+P}$ | $\dfrac{1}{4(2+P)}$ |
| $+b$ | $\dfrac{1-P}{4}$ | $-\dfrac{1}{4}$ | $-\dfrac{1}{1-P}$ | $\dfrac{1}{4(1-P)}$ |
| $a+$ | $\dfrac{1-P}{4}$ | $-\dfrac{1}{4}$ | $-\dfrac{1}{1-P}$ | $\dfrac{1}{4(1-P)}$ |
| $ab$ | $\dfrac{P}{4}$ | $\dfrac{1}{4}$ | $\dfrac{1}{P}$ | $\dfrac{1}{4P}$ |
| Total | $1$ | $0$ | — | $\dfrac{1+2P}{2P(2+P)(1-P)}$ |

TABLE 2.3

Derivation of $p$ and multiplier for score and information for the generalized intercross

| Cross | $P$ | $p$ | Score multiplier | Information multiplier |
|---|---|---|---|---|
| Coupling | $(1-p)^2$ | $1-\sqrt{P}$ | $-2(1-p)$ | $4P$ |
| Repulsion | $p^2$ | $\sqrt{P}$ | $2p$ | $4P$ |
| Mixed phase | $p(1-p)$ | $\dfrac{1-\sqrt{(1-4P)}}{2}$ | $1-2p$ | $1-4P$ |

Table 2.2 shows a similar analysis for the intercross. This analysis is illustrative of a simple device for reducing the algebraic complexity. The intercross may occur in three phases (viz., coupling, repulsion, and mixed phase) and it is possible to express all of the class expectations in terms of an ancillary parameter $P$, $P$ being a function of $p$ and differing for each of the three phases. The analysis is then conducted for $P$, resulting in a manageable quadratic estimating formulae instead of a biquadratic. The amount of information is also found in terms of $P$. This procedure enables the three intercrosses to be analysed at one time. The crossover fraction for a particular intercross is subsequently found from $P$ as summarized in Table 2.3. For example, given $P$ from a coupling intercross, $p = 1 - \sqrt{P}$.

The information per single observation for $p$ is derived by differentiating $P$ with respect to $p$. The principle is that of differentiation of a function of a function with regard to $dm/dP$. This quantity is squared and used as a multiplier to change the information for $P$ into that for $p$. The three multipliers are shown in the final column of Table 2.3. Thus, the information for the coupling intercross in terms of $p$ is:

$$4P \cdot \frac{1+2P}{2P(2+P)(1-P)} = \frac{2(1+2P)}{(2+P)(1-P)}.$$

The variance of $p$ found from the above by multiplying by $n$ and inversion in the usual way:

$$V = \frac{(2+P)(1-P)}{2n(1+2P)}.$$

The above illustrations are indicative that all (or most) of the conceivable genetic situations could be formally analysed and solved in terms of deviation of estimating formula and variance once and for all. This task is undertaken for a wide variety of situations in succeeding chapters.

When several groups of data are available, a combinational or mean value of $p$ can be obtained by weighting the individual estimates by the respective amounts of information:

$$\bar{p} = \frac{\Sigma pI}{\Sigma I}.$$

## SEVERAL PARAMETERS

For several parameters, $p$, $u$, $v$ ..., the $L$ function is differentiated successively with respect to $p$, $u$, $v$, .... Estimating functions are derived:

$$\frac{dL}{dp} = \Sigma \left( \frac{1}{m} \frac{dm}{dp} \right)$$

$$\frac{dL}{du} = \Sigma \left( \frac{1}{m} \frac{dm}{du} \right)$$

$$\frac{dL}{dv} = \Sigma \left( \frac{1}{m} \frac{dm}{dv} \right)$$

$$. . . . .$$

These functions are multiplied class by class by the corresponding observed frequency, summed, and equated to zero. The procedure follows that for a single parameter except that the resultant equations are to be treated as simultaneous equations and solved for $p$, $u$, $v$, .... For two parameters, this can usually be accomplished fairly easily. For three parameters, the algebra can be tedious but can often be lightened by the following corollary. When the number of parameters equals the number of degrees of freedom, the expectations may be equated to the observations:

$$m_1 = a$$
$$\ldots\ldots$$
$$m_t = t.$$

and solved directly (Bailey, 1949b, 1951). This condition is met by four class genetic situations and three unknowns. The resultant set of equations are often of easier solution than the maximum likelihood estimators.

Since the parameters are frequently not independent, the information functions have to be arranged as a matrix. In addition to the usual derivative equations of the form:

$$A = \sum \left[ \frac{1}{m} \left( \frac{dm}{dp} \right)^2 \right],$$

$$D = \sum \left[ \frac{1}{m} \left( \frac{dm}{du} \right)^2 \right],$$

$$F = \sum \left[ \frac{1}{m} \left( \frac{dm}{dv} \right)^2 \right],$$
$$\ldots\ldots$$

there will be others of the form:

$$B = \sum \left[ \frac{1}{m} \frac{dm}{dp} \frac{dm}{du} \right],$$

$$C = \sum \left[ \frac{1}{m} \frac{dm}{dp} \frac{dm}{dv} \right],$$

$$E = \sum \left[ \frac{1}{m} \frac{dm}{du} \frac{dm}{dv} \right],$$
$$\ldots\ldots$$

for all possible different combinations of $p, u, v \ldots$. These latter are easily built up by systematic arrangement of $m$, $dm/dp$, $dm/du$, $dm/dv \ldots$ and multiplying these appropriately over all classes.

The matrix is:

$$|A| = \begin{vmatrix} A & B & C & \cdot \\ B & D & E & \cdot \\ C & E & F & \cdot \\ \cdot & \cdot & \cdot & \cdot \end{vmatrix}$$

Let $A_{rs}$ be the signed minor of the matrix obtained by suppressing the $r$th row and $s$th column; then the variances and covariances $(CV)$ are given by:

$$V_{rs} = \frac{A_{rs}}{n\Delta}, \qquad \text{when } r = s$$

$$CV_{rs} = \frac{A_{rs}}{n\Delta}, \qquad \text{when } r \neq s$$

found by inverting $|A|$, and $\Delta$ being the determinant of $|A|$.

In the context of genetic linkage, the two recurring information matrices are the 2 x 2 and 3 x 3. The 2 x 2 matrix:

$$\begin{vmatrix} A & B \\ B & D \end{vmatrix}$$

upon inversion, becomes:

$$V_p = \frac{D}{n\Delta}, \qquad V_u = \frac{A}{n\Delta}, \qquad CV_{pu} = \frac{B}{n\Delta}$$

where $\Delta = AD - B^2$.

The 3 x 3 matrix:

$$\begin{vmatrix} A & B & C \\ B & D & E \\ C & E & F \end{vmatrix}$$

upon inversion, becomes:

$$V_p = \frac{DF - E^2}{n\Delta}, \qquad V_u = \frac{AF - C^2}{n\Delta}, \qquad V_v = \frac{AD - B^2}{n\Delta},$$

$$CV_{pu} = -\frac{BF - CE}{n\Delta}, \quad CV_{pv} = \frac{BE - CD}{n\Delta}, \qquad CV_{uv} = -\frac{AE - CB}{n\Delta}.$$

where $\Delta = A(DF - E^2) + B(CE - BF) + C(BE - CD)$.

Note, should all of the covariances equal zero, the variances become the reciprocals of their respective amounts of information, which is the case for the single parameter.

An upper limit to the number of parameters which may be estimated is set by the number of degrees of freedom. For the ordinary four-class Mendelian segregations, not more than three parameters can be estimated. By combining different segregations, the number of degrees of freedom and the number of estimable parameters can be increased. Care should be exercised, however, that it is possible to estimate the full potential number. It may be that the formulated expectations or the estimating formulae are not functionally independent. This is usually revealed by the information matrix becoming singular. Inversion, and thus estimation, is impossible.

Bailey (1951) has stressed that, in doubtful situations, the information matrix of a set of $s$ estimating formulae should be checked for non-singularity. The matrix should be examined for rank and if this is less than $s$, say $r$, then only $r$ of the estimating formulae are functionally independent. The situation should be re-cast algebraically so that $r$ parameters can be estimated (if this is possible) or the design of the experiment be suitably extended to bring in more degrees of freedom.

When several groups of data are available, mean values of $p$, $u$, $v$, . . . , can be obtained by weighting the individual estimates by the reciprocal of the respective variances:

$$\bar{p} = \frac{\Sigma p V_p^{-1}}{\Sigma V_p^{-1}},$$

$$\bar{u} = \frac{\Sigma u V_u^{-1}}{\Sigma V_u^{-1}},$$

$$\bar{v} = \frac{\Sigma v V_v^{-1}}{\Sigma V_v^{-1}}.$$

### SCORES

Wherever possible, the estimating formula:

$$\frac{\mathrm{d}L}{\mathrm{d}p} - \Sigma\left(\frac{a}{m}\frac{\mathrm{d}m}{\mathrm{d}p}\right) = 0,$$

should be solved in terms of the class frequencies. However, this may result in a polynomial in which the roots cannot be easily found. A comparatively late development has been the introduction of maximum likelihood scores to deal with the problem (Fisher, 1946; Rao, 1948, 1950, 1952).

With a single parameter, the procedure is to set up the estimating formula in the usual way but to evaluate the equation term by term by insertion of a provisional value of $p$, say $p'$. The equation will then, in general, not be equal to zero. Instead, it will yield a quantity which is defined as the score:

$$S = \sum \left( \frac{a}{m} \frac{dm}{dp'} \right),$$

where $a$ is a generalized symbol for the observed frequencies $a$, $b$, $c$, . . . .

The amount of information is also calculated for the provisional value. The score and information are then used to yield a correction factor $(\delta p)$:

$$\delta p = \frac{S}{I} = SV.$$

which is added to $p'$, with due regard to sign, to give an improved value of $p$. The cycle of calculation is repeated with successive values of $p$ until $\delta p$ has been reduced to negligibility.

With several parameters, the procedure is the same except that provisional values for each of the parameters are to be fitted into the estimating formulae to yield scores $S_p$, $S_u$, $S_v$, . . . . The information matrix, variances, and covariances are computed for the provisional values, from which the correction factors are found as:

$$\delta p = S_p V_v + S_u CV_{pu} + S_v CV_{pv} + \ldots$$
$$\delta u = S_p CV_{pu} + S_u V_u + S_v CV_{uv} + \ldots$$
$$\delta v = S_p CV_{pv} + S_u CV_{uv} + S_v V_{vv} + \ldots$$
$$\cdot \; \cdot \; \cdot \; \cdot \; \cdot$$

paying particular attention to signs.

These corrections are added to the provisional values and the cycle of calculations repeated. It is wise to choose provisional values reasonably close to the probable value (by appraising part of the data, for example). The matrix elements do not, as a rule, change so quickly as the parameters, hence the matrix need not be recalculated should it be necessary to run several cycles. When the correction factors have been reduced to negligible quantities, the values of $p$, $u$, $v$, ... are inserted for a final calculation.

One of the most useful attributes of scoring is that the technique permits of a simple, yet powerful, analysis of heterogeneity between data. Suppose that a value of $p$ is expected on theoretical grounds. This may be inserted into the usual formula to produce a score $S$. If the data were a perfect fit to expectation, $S = 0$, but $S$ will more usually differ from zero due to sampling variation. This aspect may be examined directly because:

$$\chi^2 = \frac{S^2}{I},$$

for one degree of freedom. Summation of individual $\chi^2$ over $k$ samples yields a $\chi^2$ for $k$ degrees of freedom. The scores and information for the $k$ samples can be summed and a $\chi^2$ for one degree of freedom calculated for the total. Subtraction of this $\chi^2$ for the total from the sum of the individual $\chi^2$ gives a heterogeneity $\chi^2$ for $k-1$ degrees of freedom. If the data are of a hierarchal nature, with meaningful sub-divisions, the heterogeneity analysis can take these into account.

The scoring technique can be equally well employed for a heterogeneity analysis based on an estimated mean value of $p$. The mean value of $p$ can be found with scoring as:

$$\delta \bar{p} = \frac{\Sigma S}{\Sigma I}.$$

The arithmetic is heavier than by weighting with the amount of information per individual item because of the necessity for the mean correction factor to be negligible. The sum of the scores for the individual groups of data will scarcely differ from zero and the calculated individual $\chi^2$ values will be due entirely to heterogeneity, having a total of $k-1$ degrees of freedom.

### 'REALIZED' INFORMATION

The calculation of scores enables a rapid approximation to be made for the amount of information. The approximation can be made for estimation of either a single parameter or several parameters. The most advantage to be gained would be for the latter situation, since the matrix operations are by-passed.

The amount of information is based upon the rate of change of $p$. In the case of a single parameter, this can be estimated by direct calculation of two sufficiently close scores (say, $p_1$ and $p_2$) of opposite sign:

$$I = \frac{|S_1 - S_2|}{|p_1 - p_2|}.$$

The interval between $p$'s should not be greater than 0.01. The estimated value of $p$ is found by the usual correction factor, based upon one of the above $p$'s.

In the case of several parameters, the procedure is similar except that allowance must be made for the influence of the parameters upon each other. Values of $p, u, v, \ldots$ are found by the explicit estimating formulae. Two scores of opposite sign are calculated for $p$ (say) by appropriate choice of $p$ and the insertion of the estimates for $u, v, \ldots$. The approximation is then:

$$I_p = \frac{|S_{p_1} - S_{p_2}|}{|p_1 - p_2|}.$$

A distinction is made between the expected and the realized amount of information contained in a sample. The maximum likelihood manipulations produce an estimate based upon the product of the class expectations and number in sample. The approximate calculations described above, on the other hand, are based on the observed class frequencies and represent the information actually realized. The two estimates should not differ greatly, provided the observed frequencies do not depart significantly from their expectations.

# CHAPTER 3

# Inviability, Impenetrance and Linkage Detection

The study of linkage has two phases: (a) the detection of linkage among segregating genes and (b) estimation of its strength. The two phases are certainly not distinct, except in a formal sense, for the second arises naturally from a positive answer to the first. It is self-evident that at least two mutant non-allelic genes are necessary for linkage analysis and the first question which must be answered is whether or not the genes conform to the classical Mendelian ratios. That is, to the 1 : 1 or 3 : 1 ratio of a recessive gene for the testcross or intercross generation. Regardless of the presence of other genes or of linkage, each gene should occur individually in these ratios and each should be specially checked. Those genes which conform to expectation are the most useful for extended studies and, where a choice can be exercised, should be utilized.

Disturbances of the expected ratio are due usually to one of two causes. These are inviability (partial viability) or impenetrance (partial penetrance) of the phenotype. For purposes of estimation, it is important to know which of these possibilities are operating. Fortunately, this is often evident from inspection. In the case of inviability, the survivors usually show signs of either general or specific debility, while impenetrance is frequently accompanied by variable expression of the character under consideration.

The most useful distribution for undertaking tests of significance of genetic data is the $\chi^2$. The $\chi^2$ is of extraordinary versatility and is particularly suited for the analysis of frequency data. The only precautions to be observed are not to confuse the relevant number of degrees of freedom and not to undertake tests where the expected numbers in some classes are low. The usual advice is not to proceed with a $\chi^2$ test should the expectation in one or more classes be less than five. This is sound advice, no doubt, but cognizance should also be taken of the overall situation and, in this respect, Cochran (1954) has made some pertinent comments.

The general formula for the calculation of $\chi^2$ is:

$$\chi^2 = \sum \frac{(a-mn)^2}{mn} = \sum \frac{a^2}{(mn)} - n.$$

Where $a$ is a generalized symbol for the number of observations for successive classes $(a, b, c, \ldots)$, $mn$ the expected number in each class, and $n$ the total number of observations. The two formulae are identical (Mather, 1946) but some people prefer one to the other. The right-hand formula is slightly easier to compute. When the test is simply that of comparing differences between observation and expectation, the $\chi^2$ has degrees of freedom (df) one less than the number of classes. The significance of the calculated $\chi^2$ is ascertained by reference to a $\chi^2$ table such as given by Fisher and Yates (1953).

The above expression may be used to check the assortment of an incompletely dominant gene. However, most genes display recessivity so that two class segregations are the typical situation. A simpler expression may be employed for these cases:

$$\chi^2 = \frac{(a-Rb)^2}{Rn},$$

where $R$ is the ratio of the $a : b$ classes. The ratio $\chi^2$, as it may be termed, has one df. By setting $R = 1$ or 3, respectively, genes assorting in either of the 1 : 1 or 3 : 1 ratios can be tested for agreement with the expected frequencies.

The ratio formula is of wide applicability in genetics. A later section will demonstrate that it can be extended to examine the assortment of several simultaneous genes and to take account of associations between pairs of genes. Before leaving the subject of two class segregations, however, a further application of the formula may be noted. Segregations involving more than one gene but which reduce to two classes (as a consequence of epistatic or complementary gene action) can be conveniently handled by the formula. For example, two class segregations in which the classes occur in the ratios 9 : 7, 13 : 3, or 15 : 1 can be tested by taking $R$ as equal to 15, 9/7, and 13/3, respectively.

Once either inviability or impenetrance has been shown to be associated with the assortment of a particular gene, it is desirable to assess its magnitude. Tables 3.1 and 3.2 present formulae for estimating the viability ($v$) and penetrance ($\alpha$) for a number of commonly encountered situations. The most frequent in the case of inviability is probably the first in which the recessive class is significantly deficient. Strictly, to apply the comparable estimating formula for a dominant gene which confers inviability upon its recipients, it is necessary to assume that the homozygous ($AA$) and heterozygous ($A+$) genotypes have equal mortality. A comparison of the estimated viabilities for the backcross and intercross should disclose if this assumption is false although fairly large samples may be necessary to reveal significant differences.

The two final formulae of Table 3.1 are given as a warning not to take all data to much for granted. An $F_2$ may show a

TABLE 3.1

Estimation of viability

| Situation | Estimator | Variance |
|---|---|---|
| $a$ inviable for ratio $+ : a : : R : 1$ | $\dfrac{Rb}{a}$ | $\dfrac{v(R+v)^2}{Rn}$ |
| $A$ inviable for ratio $A : + : : R : 1$ | $\dfrac{a}{Rb}$ | $\dfrac{v(Rv+1)^2}{Rn}$ |
| $AA$ inviable in $F_2$ | $\dfrac{a-2b}{b}$ | $\dfrac{(2+v)(3+v)^2}{n}$ |
| $AA$ and $++$ inviable relative to $A+$ | $\dfrac{2b}{a-b}$ | $\dfrac{v(2+v)(1+v)^2}{n}$ |

shortage of the dominant class and the deficiency could be due to preferential death of the homozygotes $AA$, the $A+$ class of being of normal viability. On the other hand, the apparent shortage of the recessive class could arise from the superiority of the heterozygote over both homozygous classes. If $v$ is assumed to represent the mean viability of the $++$ and $aa$ genotypes, then the formula of the table can be used. An alternative view would be to postulate a 'heterotic effect' $(h; h > 1)$, peculiar to $A+$, and calculate:

$$h = \frac{a-b}{2b}, \qquad V = \frac{(1+2h)(1+h)^2}{n}.$$

Impenetrance is tackled very similarly to the foregoing but because the underlying cause is different, the estimating formulae and variances are different. Table 3.2 lists formulae for the more common situations. The first and second formulae cover the cases of a recessive and dominant impenetrant gene. The final formula treats the not impossible situation of a dominant gene $A$ which attains regular expression when homozygous $(AA)$ but fails to do so for all individuals when heterozygous $(A+)$. As a consequence, some $A+$ individuals resemble $++$ in appearance.

The present discussion serves to systemize the treatment of inviability and impenetrance but, above all, to introduce these

TABLE 3.2

Estimation of penetrance

| Situation | Estimator | Variance |
|---|---|---|
| $a$ impenetrant for ratio $+ : a :: R : 1$ | $\frac{(R+1)b}{n}$ | $\frac{\alpha(R+1-\alpha)}{n}$ |
| $A$ impenetrant for ratio $A : + :: R : 1$ | $\frac{(R+1)a}{Rn}$ | $\frac{\alpha[R(1-\alpha)+1]}{Rn}$ |
| $A+$ class mimics $++$ | $\frac{3a-b}{2n}$ | $\frac{(1+2\alpha)(3-2\alpha)}{2n}$ |

factors explicitly so that their influence can be appreciated and allowed for in the calculation of crossover values. Whenever either of these factors are thought to be relevant, the usual formulae for estimating the crossover value would be only an approximation at best and could be misleading.

In most instances, the detection of linkage can be accomplished by an extension of the procedure for testing individual genes for agreement with expectation. The simultaneous segregation of two genes $a$ and $b$ produces the four phenotypes $++$, $+b$, $a+$, and $ab$. Let these occur with the frequencies $a$, $b$, $c$, and $d$. If gene $a$ was being tested, application of the ratio $\chi^2$ would require the class frequencies $a$ and $b$, and $c$ and $d$, to be pooled. Namely,

$$\chi_a^2 = \frac{[(a+b)-R_a(c+d)]^2}{R_a n} = \frac{(a+b-R_a c-R_a d)^2}{R_a n}.$$

Similarly, testing the assortment of gene $b$ produces the analogous formula:

$$\chi_b^2 = \frac{[(a+c)-R_b(b+d)]^2}{R_b n} = \frac{(a-R_b b+c-R_b d)^2}{R_b n}.$$

$R_a$ and $R_b$ represent the ratio of $+:a$ and $+:b$ expectations, respectively, of the two genes. This means that the formulae have generality in that they can be used for both the testcross and intercross by setting $R_a = R_b = 1$ or $R_a = R_b = 3$, respectively. The single backcross can be accommodated by setting $R_a = 3$ and $R_b = 1$ or $R_a = 1$ and $R_b = 3$ as the occasion demands.

The formula for detecting linkage is:

$$\chi_l^2 = \frac{(a-R_b b-R_a c+R_a R_b d)^2}{R_a R_b n}.$$

Examination of $\chi_l^2$ reveals that it is formed by cross multiplication of the $R$ coefficients of the respective class frequencies, taking note of signs. This is the principle, although certain rules have to be obeyed in the build up of the formula (Mather, 1946, 1951). Table 3.3 shows specific formulae for three of the more important segregations.

The four class segregation produced by bigenic assortment yields a $\chi^2$ with three degrees of freedom. The formulae of

Table 3.3. neatly separate this $\chi^2$ into three components, each one relevant to three sources of variation and having one df. This process may be aptly illustrated by an example. Suppose that the following intercross has been obtained $220{+}{+}$, $99{+}b$, $94a{+}$, and $15ab$. Calculation of the three $\chi^2$ 's would give:

$$\chi_a^2 = \frac{[220+99-3(94)-3(15)]^2}{3(428)} \quad = \quad 0.05$$

$$\chi_b^2 = \frac{[220-3(99)+94-3(15)]^2}{3(428)} \quad = \quad 0.61$$

$$\chi_l^2 = \frac{[220-3(99)-3(94)+3(15)]^2}{9(428)} = 13.03$$

$$\text{Total} \quad \overline{13.69}$$

The two $\chi^2$ testing assortment of the individual genes come out as insignificant while that for dependence is clearly significant. Application of the general $\chi^2$ formula to the data produces the value of 13.69 for three df, in agreement with the total found from the above $\chi^2$. This confirms that the ratio $\chi^2$ are accurately sub-dividing the total $\chi^2$.

The above example illustrates the use of the ratio formula for linkage detection in its simplest form. The single gene ratios are normal and any disturbance could only be due to chance or to linkage. Should one or more of the gene ratios be abnormal, however, the linkage component will be affected to a greater or lesser degree and should not be regarded as reliable. There are two methods of overcoming this difficulty. The first is to modify the ratio coefficients by replacing the expected ratios by those actually shown by the data. That is, calculate $R_a = (a+b)/(c+d)$ and $R_b = (a+c)/(b+d)$ and fit these in $\chi_l^2$. For convenience, it is desirable to have the coefficients greater than unity even if this means taking their reciprocals.

The second method is to employ the well-known criss-cross formula:

$$\chi^2 = \frac{(ad-bc)^2 n}{(a+b)(c+d)(a+c)(c+d)}.$$

TABLE 3.3

Detection of disturbed gene assortment and of linkage in 2-point crosses

| Cross | Expected ratios | | | | Formulae |
|---|---|---|---|---|---|
| | ++ | +b | a+ | ab | |
| Testcross | 1 | 1 | 1 | 1 | $\chi_a^2 = \dfrac{(a+b-c-d)^2}{n}$ |
| | | | | | $\chi_b^2 = \dfrac{(a-b+c-d)^2}{n}$ |
| | | | | | $\chi_l^2 = \dfrac{(a-b\ \ c+d)^2}{n}$ |
| Single backcross (a intercrossed) | 3 | 3 | 1 | 1 | $\chi_a^2 = \dfrac{(a+b-3c-3d)^2}{3n}$ |
| | | | | | $\chi_b^2 = \dfrac{(a-b+c-d)^2}{n}$ |
| | | | | | $\chi_l^2 = \dfrac{(a-b-3c+3d)^2}{3n}$ |
| Intercross | 9 | 3 | 3 | 1 | $\chi_a^2 = \dfrac{(a+b-3c-3d)^2}{3n}$ |
| | | | | | $\chi_b^2 = \dfrac{(a-3b+c-3d)^2}{3n}$ |
| | | | | | $\chi_l^2 = \dfrac{(a-3b-3c+9d)^2}{9n}$ |
| Observations | a | b | c | d | $n = a+b+c+d$ |

for one df. This $\chi^2$ analysis provides an effective check on the presence of a significant association between the phenotypes in a similar manner to $\chi_l^2$.

Even when a significant criss-cross $\chi^2$ value has been calculated it does not necessarily follow that genetic linkage is the cause. Another factor to be considered is the possibility of an interaction between the classes which may cause one or more to be present either in excess of or less than expectation. Genes producing inviable effects are apt to interact and to reduce the frequency of those classes in which they occur together. Should the joint effect be greater than the expected compound effect, then an illusion of linkage could result. The classic situation is that of a repulsion intercross with two inviable recessive genes which seriously impair the viability of the double recessive. With an adequately sized sample, the criss-cross $\chi^2$ would indicate an association between the genes but it would not be due to linkage. Independent evidence could probably provide a clue as to the nature of the interaction.

Statistically, the above situation can be tackled by means of balanced crosses in which the range of phenotypes are produced by crosses of opposition linkage phase. Estimates of the recombination fraction would be divergent and upon combination would be expected to give a value insignificantly different from that of independence.

CHAPTER 4

# Estimation with Normal Gene Ratios

Linkage is manifested whenever two simultaneously assorting genes are found to be regularly associated. In the classic Mendelian experiment, two genes should assort at random in the testcross and in the intercross. However, in some crosses, completely random assortment is not realized. In each of the crosses, the four phenotypes can be represented as formed from the original and parental combinations or as recombinations. Formally, linkage is indicated whenever the expected number of parental phenotypes significantly exceeds the expected number of recombinant phenotypes. Two linkage phases can be defined, depending upon the nature of the initial cross. Two genes are said to be in coupling or repulsion phase, according to whether they were contributed by the same or different parents.

Estimation of the strength of linkage, defined as the proportion of recombinant gametes, is best performed by the method of maximum likelihood, formal details of which are given earlier. In this, and several succeeding chapters, the expectations for many of the various types of matings and crosses will be discussed; together with the derived formula for estimating the crossover value and its large sample variance. As usual, the standard error is invariably $\sqrt{V}$.

The most direct and efficient cross for two fully dominant genes is the testcross. The expectations are, taking into account the phase of linkage:

|  | $++$ | $+b$ | $a+$ | $ab$ | Total |
|---|---|---|---|---|---|
| Coupling | $\dfrac{1-p}{2}$ | $\dfrac{p}{2}$ | $\dfrac{p}{2}$ | $\dfrac{1-p}{2}$ | 1 |

43

| Repulsion | $\dfrac{p}{2}$ | $\dfrac{1-p}{2}$ | $\dfrac{1-p}{2}$ | $\dfrac{p}{2}$ | 1 |
|---|---|---|---|---|---|
| Observations | $a$ | $b$ | $c$ | $d$ | $n$ |

Whence:

| Coupling | $p = \dfrac{a+d}{n}$, | $V = \dfrac{p(1-p)}{n}$. |
|---|---|---|
| Repulsion | $p = \dfrac{b+c}{n}$, | $V = \dfrac{p(1-p)}{n}$. |

The four phenotypic classes can be divided into those formed from non-crossover and crossover gametes. The basically simple nature of the double backcross leads to almost self-evident estimation formulae for $p$. This aspect should encourage the non-mathematical biologist to have confidence in the formulae which follow, for few others have this property. Apart from the decided simplicity of the calculations, an advantage of the testcross is that it enables an estimate to be made of $p$ for each sex.

Expectations for the two usual intercrosses may be written as:

| $++$ | $+b$ | $a+$ | $ab$ |
|---|---|---|---|
| $\dfrac{2+P}{4}$ | $\dfrac{1-P}{4}$ | $\dfrac{1-P}{4}$ | $\dfrac{P}{4}$ |

where $P = (1-p)^2$ for coupling and $p^2$ for repulsion phase. Whence:

$$P = \frac{A + \sqrt{(A^2 + 8dn)}}{2n}, \qquad V = \frac{(2+P)(1-P)}{2n(1+2P)},$$

where $A = a - 2b - 2c - d$. The crossover fraction $p$ is found from $P$ as follows: $p = 1 - \sqrt{P}$ and $p = \sqrt{P}$ for coupling and repulsion, respectively (Table 2.3). The variance formula relates to $p$, not $P$. Ordinarily, it is impossible to have separate estimates of $p$ for the sexes from an intercross. It is usual tacitly to assume that crossingover is approximately equal for each sex.

If a difference does exist, the intercross will provide an estimate of the geometric mean.

A third intercross may be noted, although it rarely occurs in experimental breeding. This is the mixed phase intercross where one parent is in coupling and the other is in repulsion. The expectations in terms of $P$ are as above but $P$ is now equal to $p(1-p)$. $P$ may be estimated by the above formula; whence $p = [1 - \sqrt{(1-4P)}]/2$.

The variance is:

$$V = \frac{2P(2+P)(1-P)}{n(1+2P)(1-4P)}.$$

This will be the only example of a mixed phase intercross although it is apparent that any of the other intercrosses to be discussed could be of this nature. In any of these cases, once $P$ has been found $p$ can be derived by the relation described above. In each instance, the variance for either the orthodox coupling or repulsion intercross must be multiplied by:

$$\frac{4P}{1-4P},$$

to give the variance for the mixed phase.

A few cautionary remarks on the intercross may not be out of place. The desirability of obtaining an adequate sample is obvious although what constitutes an adequate sample is not always immediately obvious. However, it is particularly advisable to be wary of segregations in which one or more classes have only a few representatives. Admittedly, this would indicate a low crossover value but unless a fair number of crossover types per class are recorded, the estimated value will not be reliable. The recognition of this sort of error is particularly urgent with intercross segregations in repulsion. With this sort of segregation, the addition of a single observation to a sparsely represented double recessive class can make an appreciable difference to the crossover value. Statistically, the reason is that the estimation is non-linear, being dependent upon the simultaneous occurrence of two rare events.

A repulsion intercross of adequate size but devoid of individuals of the double recessive class presents a problem. The above formula in this situation will give a zero value even if the other frequencies may hint that a low rate of crossingover had occurred. In principle, an estimate of $p$ could be derived from the expectation for the first three classes:

$$
\begin{array}{ccc}
++ & +b & a+ \\[6pt]
\dfrac{2+P}{4-P} & \dfrac{1-P}{4-P} & \dfrac{1-P}{4-P}
\end{array}
$$

Whence: $\qquad p = \dfrac{2a - 2(b+c)}{2a + b + c}, \qquad V = \dfrac{(2+P)(1-P)(4-P)^2}{18n}.$

In practice, however, this formula is not particularly reliable, due to the fact that the three classes approximate to the ratio $2 : 1 : 1$ for a low crossover value; in fact, should $b+c > a$ by sampling deviation, estimation is impossible.

If one of the genes is a newly discovered recessive, the testcross is ruled out because of the absence of the double recessive. The best procedure in the circumstance is to cross the two singly dominant classes of the non-productive intercross with each other: $+b$ x $a+$. These two classes could consist of two genotypes; either $++bb$ or $+abb$ and $aa++$ or $aa+b$. The second genotype in each case will have arisen as a single crossover. This cross performs two functions; it should produce double recessive offspring (unless the two genes are effectively alleles) necessary for the more desirable backcross and it will give an estimate of the crossover value. The cross will be simultaneously testing the $+b$ phenotype for heterozygosity for $a$ and $a+$ for heterozygosity for $b$. Hence, both parents are contributing information and the sample size will consist of the total number of different parents. If, for some reason, only one of the classes can be tested (either $+b$ or $a+$), the sample number will consist only of these animals. Supposing it is possible to detect all of the heterozygotes and grouping $aa++$ with $++bb$ and $aa+b$ with $+abb$, the expectations are

$$
\begin{array}{cc}
++bb & +abb \\[6pt]
\dfrac{1-p}{1+p} & \dfrac{2p}{1+p}
\end{array}
$$

Observations $\qquad\qquad\quad a \qquad\qquad\qquad b$

Whence: $\qquad p = \dfrac{b}{2a+b}, \qquad V = \dfrac{p(1-p)(1+p)^2}{2n}.$

A factor which must be taken into account is that some +abb and aa +b individuals may be missed because these have not produced any aa or bb young by chance. To mitigate this possibility, it is common practice to count only those parents which have produced more than a certain number of progeny, say six. The only advantage of this method is its simplicity. It would be better to utilize all of the data to hand. The larger the progeny, the smaller the chance of not recovering the appropriate recessive, should the parent be an heterozygote, according to the sequence $(0.5)^j$; where $j$ is the number of progeny. The efficiency of a particular mating may be represented by $1-(0.5)^j$. Summing these terms will give the equivalent number of fully tested parents. This total will be less than the actual number of parents but will compensate for the non-detection of a small number of heterozygotes. This principle was enunciated by Falconer (1949) in another connection and adapted by Carter (1951). Falconer describes a simple means of allowing for reduced expectation should one of the mutants be inviable or impenetrant.

Weighting each parent with $1-(0.5)^k$ means that all of the parents can be utilized although those with small progenies will not make much of a contribution. If the progeny size do not vary very much, a mean progeny size may be assumed for all (or batches of) parents, thus reducing the arithmetical work with a small sacrifice in accuracy. Table 4.1 should facilitate this work.

TABLE 4.1

Table of $1-(015)^j$

| $j$ | $1-(0.5)^j$ | $j$ | $1-(0.5)^j$ |
|---|---|---|---|
| 1 | 0.5 | 11 | 0.99951 |
| 2 | 0.75 | 12/ | 0.99976 |
| 3 | 0.875 | 13 | 0.99988 |
| 4 | 0.9375 | 14 | 0.99994 |
| 5 | 0.96875 | 15 | 0.99997 |
| 6 | 0.98438 | 16 | 0.99998 |
| 7 | 0.99219 | 17 | 0.99999 |
| 8 | 0.99609 | 18 | 1 |
| 9 | 0.99805 | 19 | 1 |
| 10 | 0.99903 | 20 | 1 |

The method was employed by Gates (1927, 1928a) and Snell (1928) in their investigation of the extremely close linkage of $d$ and $se$ in the house mouse. Gates tested a total of 202 intercross mice and failed to discover a single heterozygote. Snell had to test a far larger number (579) before a single heterozygote was found.

The single backcross is not employed as frequently as the above crosses but it has its usefulness. Taking gene $a$ as intercrossed and $b$ as backcrossed (i.e., $+a+b \times +abb$), the expectations are:

|  | $++$ | $+b$ | $a+$ | $ab$ |
|---|:---:|:---:|:---:|:---:|
| Coupling | $\dfrac{2-p}{2}$ | $\dfrac{1+p}{2}$ | $\dfrac{p}{2}$ | $\dfrac{1-p}{2}$ |
| Repulsion | $\dfrac{1+p}{2}$ | $\dfrac{2-p}{2}$ | $\dfrac{1-p}{2}$ | $\dfrac{p}{2}$ |

Whence:

Coupling    $np^3 - (3b + 2c + d)p^2 - (a - 2b + c + 2d)p + 2c = 0,$

Repulsion    $np^3 - (3a + c + 2d)p^2 - (2a - b - 2c - d)p + 2d = 0,$

and      $V = \dfrac{2(2-p)(1+p)(1-p)p}{n(1+2(1-p)p)}$     in both cases.

These cubic equations can be solved by Newton's method or fairly simply by the analogous method of scoring. A provisional estimate can be obtained from the last two classes: For coupling $p' = c/(c+d)$ and for repulsion $p' = c/(c+d)$. An appropriate score $(S)$ may be calculated from one of the following:

Coupling    $S = -\dfrac{a}{2-p} + \dfrac{b}{1+p} + \dfrac{c}{p} - \dfrac{d}{1-p},$

Repulsion    $S = \dfrac{a}{1+p} - \dfrac{b}{2-p} - \dfrac{c}{1-p} + \dfrac{d}{p},$

fitting $p'$ into the secessive terms. Each term is then multiplied by corresponding observed frequency and summed to give the score. A provisional variance is found by inserting $p'$ into the variance formulae. Since $p'$ will almost certainly differ slightly from the true value of $p$, $S$ will differ from zero. The correction factor is found as $SV$. That is:

$$p = p' + SV.$$

The cycle of calculations is repeated as many times as necessary to reduce $SV$ to a negligible quantity.

The single backcross has advantages where one of the genes is lethal or sterile, or where the double recessive is serverely inviable. In these circumstances, testcrosses are ruled out and it may be difficult to make up coupling intercrosses. The single backcross also presents a means of obtaining crossover values for each sex which might not otherwise be possible or inordinately difficult.

The analysis of segregations with incompletely dominant genes has not received much attention and this needs rectifying in view of the increasing interest being shown in codominant electrophoretic and immunogenetic variants. Advisedly, the most convenient analysis with these genes would be those crosses which stimulate testcrosses. The codominance allows classification of the offspring into non-recombinant and recombinant classes for segregations which would not usually be regarded as testcrosses. The criterion is whether the above two classes are expected to occur in equal numbers in the absence of linkage. The existence of these crosses is convenient because the statistical estimation of the crossover value from an intercross with codominant genes is not as straightforward as in the case of the ordinary intercross.

The expectations for the coupling intercross in which one of the genes is recessive $(a)$ and the other is codominant $(B$ versus $b)$ are:

| $+BB$ | $+Bb$ | $+bb$ | $aBB$ | $aBb$ | $abb$ |
|---|---|---|---|---|---|
| $\dfrac{1-p^2}{4}$ | $\dfrac{2-2p(1-p)}{4}$ | $\dfrac{p(2-p)}{4}$ | $\dfrac{p^2}{4}$ | $\dfrac{2p(1-p)}{4}$ | $\dfrac{(1-p)^2}{4}$ |
| $a$ | $b$ | $c$ | $d$ | $e$ | $f$ |

The estimating formula for $p$ would be an equation of the ninth degree and best method of finding the relevant root is by the calculation of a score and correction factor. The score is:

$$S = -\frac{2ap}{1-p^2} - \frac{b(1-2p)}{1-p(1-p)} + \frac{2c(1-p)}{p(2-p)} + \frac{2d}{p} + \frac{e(1-2p)}{p(1-p)} - \frac{2f}{1-p}.$$

The variance is found by taking the reciprocal of the information:

$$I = n\left(\frac{p^2}{1-p^2} + \frac{(1-2p)^2}{2(1-(1-p)p)} + \frac{(1-p)^2}{p(2-p)} + \frac{1}{2(1-p)p}\right).$$

A provisional value for $p$ can be found from the last three classes:

$$p' = \frac{2d-e}{2(d+e+f)}.$$

This value is used to calculate $S$ and $V$ which, in turn, produces the correction factor $SV$ or $S/I$. Unless the correction factor is satisfactorily small, $SV$ or $S/I$ is added to $p'$ and the cycle of calculations is repeated with the new value.

When the intercross is of repulsion phase, $(1-p)$ should be substituted for $p$ throughout the terms of the expectation and of $S$. The score will now take the form:

$$S = \frac{2a(1-p)}{p(2-p)} + \frac{b[1-2(1-p)]}{1-p(1-p)} - \frac{2cp}{1-p^2}$$

$$-\frac{2d}{1-p} - \frac{e[1-2(1-p)]}{p(1-p)} + \frac{2f}{p}.$$

The formulae for the provisional value of $p$ is slightly changed:

$$p' = \frac{e+2f}{2(d+e+f)}.$$

The information formula is unchanged.

The coupling intercross with two pairs of codominant genes has nine distinctive phenotypes. However, provided there is no evidence of inviability, or other complications, for individual genotypes, those with identical expectations can be grouped. The outcome is four classes with the following expectations for the coupling phase:

$$AABb$$

$$AaBB$$

| $AABB$ | $Aabb$ | | $AAbb$ |
|--------|--------|--------|--------|
| $aabb$ | $aaBb$ | $AaBb$ | $aaBB$ |
| $\dfrac{(1-p)^2}{2}$ | $\dfrac{4p(1-p)}{2}$ | $\dfrac{1-2p(1-p)}{2}$ | $\dfrac{p^2}{2}$ |
| $a$ | $b$ | $c$ | $d$ |

The estimating formula for $p$ is a lengthy equation of the third degree. Thus, $p$ is best found by calculating the score and correction factor. The score is:

$$S = -\frac{2a}{1-p} + \frac{b(1-2p)}{p(1-p)} - \frac{2c(1-2p)}{1-2p(1-p)} + \frac{2d}{p}.$$

and the variance:

$$V = \frac{[1-2p(1-p)]\,(1-p)p}{2n[1-3p(1-p)]}.$$

A provisional value for $p$ can be obtained from the two middle classes as follows:

$$P' = \frac{2b \pm \sqrt{[4b^2 + a(a+2b)]}}{4(a+2b)}, \qquad \text{whence } p' = \frac{1-\sqrt{(1-4P')}}{2}.$$

As before, this value is used to calculate $S$ and $V$, and thence the correction factor to realize a more accurate value for $p$.

When the intercross is of repulsion phase, $p$ and $1-p$ must be interchanged in the expectations. The score is modified to:

$$S = \frac{2a}{p} + \frac{b(1-2p)}{p(1-p)} - \frac{2c(1-2p)}{1-2p(1-p)} - \frac{2d}{1-p}.$$

Formulae for $V$ and $p'$ are unchanged.

The source of the algebraic complexity in the above crosses is due to the $AaBa$ class and, genetically, this arises because the class consists of two genotypes: namely $AB/ab$ and $Ab/aB$, differing in phase. If these two types of individual are distinguished by progeny tests, the estimation would be greatly simplified. The expectation for each genotype is $(1-p^2)/2$ and $p^2/2$ for coupling phase and these expectations are identical to the first and fourth classes of the expectations given earlier. The four class segregation, therefore, reduces to three and, if these are represented by the observed frequencies $a$, $b$, and $d$, respectively, have the expectations:

<table>
<tr><td>$a$</td><td>$b$</td><td>$d$</td></tr>
<tr><td>$\dfrac{(1-p)^2}{4}$</td><td>$\dfrac{p(1-p)}{2}$</td><td>$\dfrac{p^2}{4}$</td></tr>
</table>

Whence:

$$p = \frac{b+2d}{2n} \quad \text{and} \quad V = \frac{p(1-p)}{2n}.$$

If the intercross has been of repulsion phase, the expectations will be in the reverse order, and the estimator is:

$$p = \frac{2b+d}{2n} \quad \text{and} \quad V = \frac{p(1-p)}{2n}.$$

Under certain circumstances, it may be worth while to incur the extra trouble of progeny testing the class $c$ individuals of the original intercross in order to separate the phases. In addition to the simplified analysis and the gain in information, the $F_3$ progeny are available for further estimates of $p$ (Allard, 1956).

It is unfortunate that the analysis of the intercross with two pairs of codominant genes leads to such cumbersome algebra since this intercross yields more statistical information on $p$ than the testcross. The tedious algebra is probably not on the same level of disadvantage as the lack of discrimination of differences of crossingover between the sexes. This latter is the main reason for the preferential use of the testcross. The intercross with only one codominant gene is not superior to the testcross although it does yield more information than the intercross with two fully dominant genes.

When the homozygote of one of the alleles under test is a pre-natal lethal, several new situations make an appearance. These genes are usually dominant, so that while the homozygote (say $A'A'$) is never, or rarely seen, the heterozygote $A'+$ is phenotypically distinct from type. The usual procedure would be to make up a testcross, in which event the lethality would not enter the picture and the calculations will be those of an ordinary testcross. However, for the intercross and one of the single backcrosses, the lethality will modify the expectations.

The expectations for the coupling intercross with $A'A'$ lethal are:

| $A'+$ | $A'b$ | $++$ | $+b$ |
|---|---|---|---|
| $\dfrac{2-2p(1-p)}{3}$ | $\dfrac{2p(1-p)}{3}$ | $\dfrac{p(2-p)}{3}$ | $\dfrac{(1-p)^2}{3}$ |
| $a$ | $b$ | $c$ | $d$ |

The estimator for $p$ is an equation of the seventh degree. The crossover fraction may be found by the usual calculation of the score, the information and correction factor. The score is:

$$S = -\frac{a(1-2p)}{1-p(1-p)} + \frac{b(1-2p)}{p(1-p)} + \frac{2c(1-p)}{p(2-p)} - \frac{2d}{(1-p)},$$

and the information

$$I = \frac{2n}{3p}\left(\frac{1-4p(1-p)}{(1-p)[1-p(1-p)]} + \frac{2}{(2-p)}\right).$$

A provisional value of $p$ may be derived from the last two classes as:

$$p' = 1 - \sqrt{\frac{d}{c+d}}$$

and used in the above formulae to give the correction factor.

The procedures for the comparable repulsion intercross are identical to those above, taking into account the changes in expectations due to the reciprocal interchange of $p$ and $1-p$. The score is now:

$$S = -\frac{a(1-2p)}{1-p(1-p)} + \frac{b(1-2p)}{p(1-p)} - \frac{2cp}{1-p^2} + \frac{2d}{p}$$

and the information:

$$I = \frac{2n}{3}\left(\frac{1-4p(1-p)}{p(1-p)[1-p(1-p)]} + \frac{2}{1-p^2}\right).$$

A provisional estimate of $p$ may be found from the last two classes:

$$p' = \sqrt{\frac{d}{c+d}}.$$

In the case of the single backcross, the expectations for all types CBI and RBI will not be modified but those for CIB and RIB will be. For CIB and RIB, the phenotypes $A'+$ and $A'b$ will be composed of equal proportions of non-recombinants and recombinant genotypes and contribute no information. The other two classes will have the expectations:

|              | $++$    | $+b$    |
|--------------|---------|---------|
| Coupling     | $p$     | $1-p$   |
| Repulsion    | $1-p$   | $p$     |
| Observations | $c$     | $d$     |

Whence:

| Coupling  | $p = \dfrac{c}{c+d}$, | $V = \dfrac{p(1-p)}{c+d}$. |
|-----------|------------------------|-----------------------------|
| Repulsion | $p = \dfrac{d}{c+d}$, | $V = \dfrac{p(1-p)}{c+d}$. |

In experiments with a codominant pair of genes, the only crosses which require special attention are the intercrosses. The coupling intercross has six distinguishable phenotypic classes but, with the usual precautions, three of these may be grouped because of identical expectations. The expectations may be written:

$A'+BB$

$A'+bb$

| $++bb$               | $A'+Bb$              | $+BB$           | $abb$               |
|----------------------|----------------------|-----------------|---------------------|
| $\dfrac{6p(1-p)}{3}$ | $\dfrac{2-4p(1-p)}{3}$ | $\dfrac{p^2}{3}$ | $\dfrac{(1-p)^2}{3}$ |
| $a$                  | $b$                  | $c$             | $d$                 |

The estimating formula is a high degree polynomial, hence the scoring procedure should be adopted. The score is:

$$S = \frac{3a(1-2p)}{p(1-p)} - \frac{2b(1-2p)}{1-2p(1-p)} + \frac{2c}{p} - \frac{2d}{(1-p)}$$

and the information:

$$I = \frac{2n}{3}\left(\frac{4(1-2p)^2}{1-2p(1-p)} + \frac{1+2(1-2p)^2}{p(1-p)}\right).$$

A provisional value of $p$ may be obtained from the classes:

$$a \qquad\qquad c \qquad\qquad d$$

in the form:

$$p' = \frac{a+2c}{2(a+c+d)}.$$

The repulsion intercross has similar expectations except for the interchange of $p$ and $1-p$. Effectively, this means the simple transposition of the last two classes. The score is now:

$$S = \frac{3a(-12p)}{p(1-p)} - \frac{2b(1-2p)}{1-2p(1-p)} - \frac{2c}{(1-p)} + \frac{2d}{p}.$$

The information is the same as for the coupling intercross but the expression for a provisional estimate of $p$ is modified to:

$$p' = \frac{a+2d}{2(a+c+d)}.$$

The testing for possible linkage between two loci with lethality of their respective homozygotes (say $A'A'$ and $B'B'$) can be dealt with by one or another of the preceding formulae, with the exception of the intercrosses. The sensible procedure would be a testcross. However, the intercrosses may be briefly considered. The coupling intercross has four distinctive phenotypes but two of these have identical expectations and may be grouped for analysis. The expectations are:

| $A'B'$ | $A'+$<br>$+B'$ | $++$ |
|---|---|---|
| $\dfrac{2-4p(1-p)}{3-p(2-p)}$ | $\dfrac{4p(1-p)}{3-p(2-p)}$ | $\dfrac{(1-p)^2}{3-p(2-p)}$ |
| $a$ | $b$ | $c$ |

The estimating formula is a high degree polynomial and scoring is advisable to derive $p$. The score is:

$$S = -\frac{2a[2-p(5-p)]}{A[1-2p(1-p)]} + \frac{2b[3-p(6-p)]}{Ap(1-p)} - \frac{4c}{A(1-p)},$$

where $A = 3-p(2-p)$.

The information is:

$$I = \frac{4n}{[3-p(2-p)]^3}\left(4 + \frac{2[2-p(5-p)]^2}{1-2p(1-p)} + \frac{[3-p(6-p)]^2}{p(1-p)}\right).$$

There is no simple formula for a provisional estimate of $p$, so recourse must be made to an intelligent guess.

The repulsion intercross has similar expectations to the above, except for the usual interchange of $p$ and $1-p$. The score is:

$$S = -\frac{2a[2-p(3+p)]}{(2+p^2)[1-2p(1-p)]} + \frac{2b[2-p(4+p)]}{(2+p^2)p(1-p)} + \frac{4c}{(2+p^2)p}$$

and the information:

$$I = \frac{4n}{(2+p^2)^3}\left(4 + \frac{4[2-p(3+p)]^2}{1-2p(1-p)} + \frac{[2-p(4+p)]^2}{p(1-p)}\right).$$

As in the previous case, there is no simple formula for a provisional estimate of $p$.


### EPISTASIS AND DUPLICATION

Epistasis reduces the number of phenotypic classes but estimation of $p$ is still practical provided the classes which remain can be divided into non-recombinant and recombinant phenotypes. The efficiency of crosses involving epistasis compares poorly with those in which all of the classes are distinguishable. In general, the procedure is to ignore the epistatic classes and it is this wastage which lowers the efficiency. However, linkage tests with epistatic genes are often obligatory. A good example is that of albinism among the mammalian coat colour genes. This gene is epistatic to all other colour genes. On the other hand, certain alleles of albinism are not so totally epistatic and these should be preferably chosen in experiments with this particular locus.

The testcross is still the most convenient cross. With a recessive epistatic gene (say $a$), the usual four class segregations are reduced to two. The expectations for the distinguishable classes are:

|  | ++ | +b |
|---|---|---|
| Coupling | $1-p$ | $p$ |
| Repulsion | $p$ | $1-p$ |

Whence:

Coupling          $p = \dfrac{b}{a+b}$

$$V = \dfrac{p(1-p)}{a+b}$$

Repulsion          $p = \dfrac{a}{a+b}$

With a dominant epistatic gene at the $a$ locus, the expectations will be the reverse of the above for the same phenotypic classes. The estimates will be:

Coupling          $p = \dfrac{c}{c+d}$

$$V = \dfrac{p(1-p)}{c+d}$$

Repulsion          $p = \dfrac{d}{c+d}$

The symbols for the observed frequencies in the above formulae (and those immediately following) are the same as those for the corresponding non-epistatic segregations.

An intercross with a recessive epistatic gene will produce the $9:3:4$ ratio in the absence of linkage. Estimation will be based on the first two classes and the expectations are:

|  | ++ | +b |
|---|---|---|
|  | $\dfrac{2+P}{3}$ | $\dfrac{1-P}{3}$ |

Whence:

$$P = \frac{2b-a}{a-b}, \qquad V = \frac{(2+P)(1-P)}{4P(a+b)}.$$

GMLM-3

An intercross with a dominant epistatic gene will produce a 12 : 3 : 1 ratio in the absence of linkage and estimation will be from the last two classes. The expectations are:

$$++ \qquad\qquad +b$$

$$1-P \qquad\qquad P$$

Whence:

$$P = \frac{d}{c+d}, \qquad V = \frac{1-P}{4(c+d)},$$

$p = 1 - \sqrt{P}$ and $\sqrt{P}$ for coupling and repulsion, respectively, for the two cases. It should be noted that similar problems of obtaining a reliable estimate for $p$ will occur when the crossover rate is low. This is particularly true for the repulsion intercross as discussed previously. Again, test mating of the singly dominant class would be in order where a new recessive gene is concerned.

Single backcrosses in conjunction with either a recessive or dominant gene results in a variety of estimating formulae, depending whether or not the epistatic gene forms the intercrossing locus. These formulae, together with their variances, are set out in Table 4.2.

Epistasis may take the form in which two genes with mimicking phenotypes have to be tested for linkage. Three situations can be visualized. The most common is probably that of two recessive genes showing a common phenotype. It is probably worth while to establish a double recessive as an initial step since this means that testcrosses can be performed. For testcrosses, the expectations are:

|            | ++            | +b, a+, ab    |
|------------|---------------|---------------|
| Coupling   | $\frac{1-p}{2}$ | $\frac{1+p}{2}$ |
| Repulsion  | $\frac{p}{2}$   | $\frac{2-p}{2}$ |
| Observation | $a$           | $b$           |

Whence:

| | | |
|---|---|---|
| Coupling  | $p = \dfrac{b-a}{n},$ | $V = \dfrac{(1+p)(1-p)}{n}.$ |
| Repulsion | $p = \dfrac{2a}{n},$  | $V = \dfrac{p(2-p)}{n}.$ |

TABLE 4.2

Expectations and estimation in single backcrosses with epistasis. Locus $a$ taken as epistatic recessive or dominant

| | Locus | | Phase | Expectations | | $p$ | $V$ |
|---|---|---|---|---|---|---|---|
| | $a$ | $b$ | | $++$ | $+b$ | | |
| Rec. | I | B | C | $\dfrac{2-p}{3}$ | $\dfrac{1+p}{3}$ | $\dfrac{2b-a}{a+b}$ | $\dfrac{(1+p)(2-p)}{a+b}$ |
| Rec. | I | B | R | $\dfrac{1+p}{3}$ | $\dfrac{2-p}{3}$ | $\dfrac{2a-b}{a+b}$ | $\dfrac{(1+p)(2-p)}{a+b}$ |
| Rec. | B | I | C | $\dfrac{2-p}{2}$ | $\dfrac{p}{2}$ | $\dfrac{2b}{a+b}$ | $\dfrac{p(2-p)}{a+b}$ |
| Rec. | B | I | R | $\dfrac{1+p}{2}$ | $\dfrac{1-p}{2}$ | $\dfrac{a-b}{a+b}$ | $\dfrac{(1+p)(1-p)}{a+b}$ |
| Dom. | I | B | C | $p$ | $1-p$ | $\dfrac{c}{c+d}$ | $\dfrac{p(1-p)}{c+d}$ |
| Dom. | I | B | R | $1-p$ | $p$ | $\dfrac{d}{c+d}$ | $\dfrac{p(1-p)}{c+d}$ |
| Dom. | B | I | C | $\dfrac{1+p}{2}$ | $\dfrac{1-p}{2}$ | $\dfrac{c-d}{c+d}$ | $\dfrac{(1+p)(1-p)}{c+d}$ |
| Dom. | B | I | R | $\dfrac{2-p}{2}$ | $\dfrac{p}{2}$ | $\dfrac{2d}{c+d}$ | $\dfrac{p(2-p)}{c+d}$ |

Note: Rec. = recessive, Dom. = dominant, I = intercross, B = backcross, C = coupling, R = repulsion.

The intercross for two recessive mimicking genes produces the familiar 9 : 7 ratio in the absence of linkage, for which the expectations are:

| ++ | +b, a+, ab |
|----|-----------|
| $\dfrac{2+p}{4}$ | $\dfrac{2-p}{4}$ |

Whence:

$$P = \frac{2(a-b)}{n}, \qquad V = \frac{(2+P)(2-P)}{4nP}.$$

A variation on the present situation is that while the $a+$ and $+b$ phenotypes may have similar phenotypes, the genes could interact to produce a distinctive phenotype for the double recessive. If the new phenotype can be reliably detected, the expectations for the two testcrosses are:

|  | ++ | +b, a+ | ab |
|--|----|--------|----|
| Coupling | $\dfrac{1-p}{2}$ | $p$ | $\dfrac{1-p}{2}$ |
| Repulsion | $\dfrac{p}{2}$ | $1-p$ | $\dfrac{p}{2}$ |
| Observation | $a$ | $b$ | $c$ |

Whence:

Coupling $\quad p = \dfrac{b}{n}$

$$V = \frac{p(1-p)}{n}$$

Repulsion $\quad p = \dfrac{a+c}{n}$

For the intercross, the effect of the interaction would be to change the 9 : 7 ratio to that of 9 : 6 : 1 in the absence of linkage. The expectations are:

| ++ | +b, a+ | ab |
|----|--------|----|
| $\dfrac{2+P}{4}$ | $\dfrac{(1-P)}{2}$ | $\dfrac{P}{4}$ |

Whence:

$$P = \frac{A + \sqrt{(A^2 + 8cn)}}{2n}, \qquad V = \frac{(2+P)(1-P)}{2n(1+2P)}.$$

Where $A = a - 2b - c$.

It may be noted that the estimating formulae and variances are identical to those of the ordinary testcross and intercross. This is so because the merging of phenotypes, due to the identicality of the $+b$ and $a+$ phenotypes, correspond to summation of these classes by the estimating formulae.

The second situation is that of a dominant and a recessive gene showing the same phenotype. The testcross can be carried out easily in this case. Defining $A'$ as the dominant gene, the expectations are:

|  | $++$ | $A'+, A'b, ab$ |
|---|---|---|
| Coupling | $\dfrac{p}{2}$ | $\dfrac{2-p}{2}$ |
| Repulsion | $\dfrac{1-p}{2}$ | $\dfrac{1+p}{2}$ |
| Observation | $a$ | $b$ |

Whence:

Coupling $\qquad p = \dfrac{2a}{n}, \qquad V = \dfrac{p(2-p)}{n}.$

Repulsion $\qquad p = \dfrac{b-a}{n}, \qquad V = \dfrac{(1+p)(1-p)}{n}.$

The intercross in this case produces the ratio $13 : 3$ in the absence of linkage. The expectations for the two classes are:

|  $A'+, A'b, +b$  |  $++$  |
|---|---|
| $\dfrac{3+P}{4}$ | $\dfrac{1-P}{4}$ |

Whence:

$$P = \frac{a-3b}{n}, \qquad V = \frac{(3+P)(1-P)}{4nP}.$$

The last situation is that of two dominant genes with the same phenotype. As before, the testcross can easily be executed, the only difference between the present situation and those described previously residing in the particular genotype classes which are indistinguishable. The expectations are:

$$A'B', A'+, B'+ \qquad ++$$

| | $A'B', A'+, B'+$ | $++$ |
|---|---|---|
| Coupling | $\dfrac{2-p}{2}$ | $\dfrac{p}{2}$ |
| Repulsion | $\dfrac{1+p}{2}$ | $\dfrac{1-p}{2}$ |

Whence:

Coupling $\qquad p = \dfrac{2b}{n}, \qquad V = \dfrac{p(2-p)}{n}.$

Repulsion $\qquad p = \dfrac{b-a}{n}, \qquad V = \dfrac{(1+p)(1-p)}{n}.$

The intercross for two dominant genes produces the ratio 15 : 1 in the absence of linkage and the expectations are:

$$A'B', A'+, +B' \qquad ++$$

| | $A'B', A'+, +B'$ | $++$ |
|---|---|---|
| | $\dfrac{4-P}{4}$ | $\dfrac{P}{4}$ |

Whence:

$$p = \frac{4b}{n}, \qquad V = \frac{4-P}{4n}.$$

## COMPLEMENTARY GENES

A character may be determined by more than one gene and it may be necessary to subject these to linkage tests with segregation of single genes. Two simplifying suppositions are commonly made. Firstly, that the complementary genes are independent of each other and, secondly, that the number of these is limited. This assumption of a limit is not merely a matter of convenience, for it is usually difficult to keep track of more than two complementary genes. The discovery of linkage for one of a pair of such genes would be a useful means of individual identification. For this reason alone, attempts to establish linkage are worth while. Two aspects will be discussed:

firstly, the estimation of linkage between the complementary genes themselves and, secondly, the estimation of linkage between one of the genes and a third, phenotypically different, gene.

The term complementary is employed to indicate genes which produce no phenotypic change when present singly but do so when both are present in the individual. That is, in terms of gene action, the genes complement each other. A large number of situations could be depicted but only the more straightforward cases will be discussed. These have been known to occur, albeit rarely, and the discussion will be instructive of how more complex situations could be treated. No attempt will be made to deal with the added complexity of inviability or impenetrance in the present context. It is easy to conceive situations where these can be a problem but—at this time at least—the importance of these cases is very marginal.

The analysis of linkage with characters determined by complementary genes has been discussed by Hutchinson (1929), Immer (1930), Bhat (1950), Murty (1954a), and Allard (1956). Bhat has described a simple method by which the phenotypic class expectations can be formulated. Murty has given a comprehensive list of situations, extending the analysis to deal with characters determined by more than two complementary genes. He even discusses the problem of linkage estimation for two characters, each of which is determined by complementary genes. The efficiency of estimation for the latter is very low indeed.

The most frequently encountered situation is probably that of two recessive genes combining to produce a mutant phenotype. In the absence of linkage, the ratio of type and mutant phenotype will be 3 : 1 and 15 : 1 for the testcross and intercross, respectively. If there is sound independent evidence for the existence of two genes, a departure from these ratios could be indicative of linkage between them. The estimation of linkage would proceed as described in the previous section for two dominant mimicking genes except that the ratio of type : mutant is now reversed. Arithmetically, this means that the type and mutant class frequencies must be interchanged; otherwise, the estimating formulae and variances for the testcross and intercross are identical.

In the following discussions, of the possibility that one of the two genes is linked to a third, it will be assumed that the complementary genes will enter the crosses together (seemingly the most realistic case) and hence will be in coupling phase. Relative to the phenotypically distinct gene, the complementary pair may be either in coupling or repulsion. Let $a$ and $b$ represent the complementary genes and $(+)$ and $(ab)$ the type and mutant phenotypes produced. Linkage with a third recessive gene $c$ will give the following expectations for the coupling backcross to the triple recessive:

| Gene | $(+)+$ | $(+)c$ | $(ab)+$ | $(ab)c$ |
|------|--------|--------|---------|---------|
| $a$ | $\dfrac{2-p}{4}$ | $\dfrac{1+p}{4}$ | $\dfrac{p}{4}$ | $\dfrac{1-p}{4}$ |
| $b$ | $\dfrac{2-p}{4}$ | $\dfrac{1+p}{4}$ | $\dfrac{p}{4}$ | $\dfrac{1-p}{4}$ |
| Observation | $a$ | $b$ | $c$ | $d$ |

Whence:

$$np^3 - (3b + 2c + d) - (a - 2b + c + 2d)p + 2c = 0,$$

$$V = \frac{2(2-p)(1+p)(1-p)p}{n[1+2(1-p)p]}.$$

The crossover fraction can be found by any of the methods for the location of the roots of a cubic equation but calculation of scores is almost as quick as any. A provisional estimate of $p$ can be derived from the last two classes as $p' = c/(c+d)$ and this value can be fitted into the score:

$$S = -\frac{a}{2-p} + \frac{b}{1+p} + \frac{c}{p} - \frac{d}{1-p}.$$

A provisional variance is also found by use of the same $p'$, whence the correction factor $SV$ is added to $p'$. If the provisional $p'$ has been well chosen, only a few cycles of calculation will be required to reduce the product $SV$ to a minute quantity. With repulsion testcrosses, the same formulae will hold, except for the substitution of the frequencies $b$ for $a$, $a$ for $b$, $d$ for $c$, and $c$ for $d$ in the estimator and score.

The intercross generation has the expectations:

| $(+)+$ | $(+)c$ | $(ab)+$ | $(ab)c$ |
|--------|--------|---------|---------|
| $\dfrac{11+P}{16}$ | $\dfrac{4-P}{16}$ | $\dfrac{1-P}{16}$ | $\dfrac{P}{16}$ |

Whence:

$$nP^3 - (5a - 10b - 7c - 6d)P^2 + (4a - 11b - 44c - 51d)P + 44d = 0,$$

$$V = \frac{(11+P)(4-P)(1-P)}{n[11+2P(1-2P)]}.$$

The score for the above cross is:

$$S = \frac{a}{11+P} - \frac{b}{4-P} - \frac{c}{1-P} + \frac{d}{P}.$$

A provisional value of $P$ may be obtained from the last two classes as $P' = d/(c+d)$. This value may be inserted into the score and into the variance to give the correction factor $SV$. This is added to $P'$ to yield a revised value. Several cycles of calculation may be required to reduce the correction factor to a negligible quantity. The crossover fraction $p$ is derived from $P$ by the usual relation according to the phase (Table 2.3).

Another situation which may occur is that of two dominant genes which can only produce a mutant phenotype when both are present in the individual. This is the reverse of the previous situation. In the absence of linkage between them, the ratio of type and mutant will be 3 : 1 and 7 : 9 for the testcross and intercross, respectively. A departure from these ratios could be indicative of linkage. In this event, the appropriate estimating formulae from the preceding section may be employed. In the case of the 7 : 9 ratio, these will be the formulae for two recessive duplicative genes but with interchange of the type and mutant classes.

Representing the two dominant complementary genes by $A'$ and $B'$ and their joint mutant phenotype by $(A'B')$, the expectations for the coupling testcross with a phenotypically different gene will be:

| Gene | $(A'B')+$ | $(A'B')c$ | $(+)+$ | $(+)c$ |
|---|---|---|---|---|
| $A'$ | $\dfrac{p}{4}$ | $\dfrac{1-p}{4}$ | $\dfrac{2-p}{4}$ | $\dfrac{1+p}{4}$ |
| $B'$ | $\dfrac{p}{4}$ | $\dfrac{1-p}{4}$ | $\dfrac{2-p}{4}$ | $\dfrac{1+p}{4}$ |

Whence:

$$np^3 - (2a+b+3d)p^2 - (a+2b+c-2d)p + 2a = 0,$$

$$V = \frac{2(2-p)(1+p)(1-p)p}{n[1+2(1-p)p]},$$

$$S = \frac{a}{p} - \frac{b}{1-p} - \frac{c}{2-p} + \frac{d}{1+p}.$$

The expectations are the same as in the previous situation but for the interchange of classes. The estimation procedure will be the same, with a provisional estimate of $p$ obtained from any convenient two of the phenotype classes. The score is slightly different but only because of the interchangeability of the class expectations. The correction factor will have the form $SV$. The repulsion phase will have the same expectation with the appropriate interchange of classes. To deal with this case, it is necessary to substitute $b$ for $a$, $a$ for $b$, $d$ for $c$, and $c$ for $d$ in the relevant formulae.

The intercross has the following expectations:

| $(A'B')+$ | $(A'B')c$ | $(+)+$ | $(+)c$ |
|---|---|---|---|
| $\dfrac{3(2+P)}{16}$ | $\dfrac{3(1-P)}{16}$ | $\dfrac{3(2-P)}{16}$ | $\dfrac{1+3P}{16}$ |

Whence:

$$3nP^3 - (8a-b-4c+3d)P^2 +$$
$$+(3a-12b-5c-12d)P + 2a-4b-2c+12d = 0,$$

$$V = \frac{(2+P)(1-P)(2-P)(1+3P)}{3P[5+2P(1-2P)]},$$

$$S = \frac{a}{2+P} - \frac{b}{1-P} - \frac{c}{2-P} + \frac{d}{1+3P}.$$

Estimation of $p$ will proceed exactly as for the testcross.

One further situation deserves consideration because the intercross has different expectations depending upon which of the two complementary genes shows linkage. This is where the complementary phenotype is dependent upon the simultaneous presence of a dominant and a recessive gene. In the absence of linkage between the pair of genes, the ratio of type and mutant will be 3 : 1 and 13 : 3 for the testcross and intercross, respectively. Any departure from this expectation could infer linkage. The appropriate estimating formulae from the preceding section should be chosen for the subsequent analysis. In the case of the intercross, this will be for formula for the dominant and recessive duplicative genes but with interchange of the type and mutant classes.

The complementary genes may be represented by $A'$ and $b$ and the mutant phenotype as $(A'b)$ in the usual way. To carry out the testcross in the present case would entail the synthesis of the triple recessive $++bbcc$ strain. Phenotypically normal (except for $c$, the testing gene) but capable of producing four distinguishable phenotypes (when the triheterozygote $A'b+/+ +c$ is testcrossed to it) with the expectations:

$$(+)+ \qquad (+)c \qquad (A'b)+ \qquad (A'b)c$$
$$\frac{1+p}{4} \qquad \frac{2-p}{4} \qquad \frac{1-p}{4} \qquad \frac{p}{4}$$

These expectations are exactly the same as in the repulsion backcross for the situation for two recessive complementary genes. The procedures of estimation of $p$ and of the calculation of the variance will be identical to this previous situation. Should linkage be discovered, the data will give no indication which of the two genes is involved.

In the case of the intercross, the different mode of inheritance of $A'$ and $b$ means that linkage with one or the other will result in different expectations. Linkage of a recessive gene with $A'$ gives the expectations:

$$(+)+ \qquad (+)c \qquad (A'b)+ \qquad (A'b)c$$
$$\frac{10-P}{16} \qquad \frac{3+P}{16} \qquad \frac{2+P}{16} \qquad \frac{1-P}{16}$$

Whence:

$$nP^3 + (4a - 9b - 8c - 5d)P^2 +$$
$$(a - 12b - 23c - 44d) - 6a + 20b + 30c - 60d = 0,$$

$$V = \frac{(10 - P)(3 + P)(2 + P)(1 - P)}{nP[29 + 2P(1 - 2P)]},$$

$$S = -\frac{a}{10 - P} + \frac{b}{3 - P} + \frac{c}{2 + P} - \frac{d}{1 - P}.$$

The estimate of $P$ and the derivation of $p$ and $V$ will proceed as for the previous situations.

Linkage of a recessive gene with the recessive component of the complementation, on the other hand, gives the expectations:

| $(+)+$ | $(+)c$ | $(A'b)+$ | $(A'b)c$ |
|---|---|---|---|
| $\dfrac{3(3 + P)}{16}$ | $\dfrac{4 - 3P}{16}$ | $\dfrac{3(1 - P)}{16}$ | $\dfrac{2P}{16}$ |

Whence:

$$3nP^3 - (7a - 6b - 5c - 2d)P^2 + (4a - 9b - 12c - 17d)P + 12 = 0,$$

$$V = \frac{(3 + P)(4 - 3P)(1 - P)P}{3n[3 + 2P(1 - 2P)]},$$

$$S = \frac{a}{3 + P} - \frac{3b}{4 - 3P} - \frac{c}{1 - P} + \frac{d}{P}.$$

The estimate of $P$ and the derivation of $p$ and $V$ will proceed as for the previous situations.

In both of the earlier situations, only one estimating forula could be derived and, when linkage is evident, there is no means of ascertaining which of the complementary genes is linked. Yet, in the third case, it is possible for a decision to be made in this respect. When linkage is foreshadowed (for example, by an initial $\chi^2$ test for agreement between observed and expected frequencies on the basis of independent assortment) the data should be analysed by both formulae and the expectations given by both should be compared with the observed class frequencies. The resulting $\chi^2$ will have two df and the formula which gives the closer fit to the observations will indicate the relevant linkage. There should be little difficulty in deciding which of the two complementary genes is showing linkage provided (a) the linkage is not too weak and (b) adequate numbers of observations are available.

The testing of a dominant gene (say $C'$) against complementary genes can be accommodated by substituting $C'$ for $+$ and $+$ for $c$ in the phenotype symbols shown to the right of the brackets. The subsequent estimation procedures are unchanged.

# CHAPTER 5

# Estimation with Inviability

A common cause of distortion of the normal Mendelian ratios is that of relative inviability. Viability is defined as the proportion of surviving individuals carrying one allele relative to another at a particular locus. Usually, this is the mutant allele in comparison to the wild type. Two situations can arise: either one or both loci of a given segregation may have alleles which are capable of inducing inviability. These situations will be discussed in turn. It is also possible for viability interactions to occur, reducing the viability of certain classes to a greater extent than that of simple proportionality. Two interesting papers on estimation with inviability are Bailey (1949a, b).

## ONE INVIABLE LOCUS

The simplest case is that of the testcross with one recessive inviable gene. Defining the $a$ locus as inviable, the expectations are:

|  | $++$ | $+b$ | $a+$ | $ab$ |
|---|---|---|---|---|
| Coupling | $\dfrac{1-p}{2}$ | $\dfrac{p}{2}$ | $\dfrac{vp}{2}$ | $\dfrac{v(1-p)}{2}$ |
| Repulsion | $\dfrac{p}{2}$ | $\dfrac{1-p}{2}$ | $\dfrac{v(1-p)}{2}$ | $\dfrac{vp}{2}$ |
| Observations | $a$ | $b$ | $c$ | $d$ |

Whence:

Coupling
$$p = \frac{b+c}{n}, \qquad V = \frac{p(1-p)}{n}.$$

70

Repulsion $$p = \frac{a+d}{n}, \qquad V = \frac{p(1-p)}{n}.$$

The interesting aspect of the present analysis is that the inviability does not enter into the estimator of $p$ nor into the variance formula. The reason is that the inviability is combined symmetrically with $p$ over all four classes. There is a fall of efficiency of estimation (relative to estimation with fully viable genes) but this occurs as reduced sample size. The formula for $v$ is $(c+d)/(a+b)$ which is comparable to that for estimating $v$ from examination of the single gene ratio.

When the inviability is due to a dominant gene at the $a$ locus (say $A'$), the above formulae are still applicable. $A'$ should be substituted for $+$ and $+$ for $a$ to give the appropriate expectations. The formula for $v = (a+b)/(c+d)$.

The expectations for an intercross with a recessive inviable gene are:

| $++$ | $+b$ | $a+$ | $ab$ |
|------|------|------|------|
| $\dfrac{2+P}{3+v}$ | $\dfrac{1-P}{3+v}$ | $\dfrac{v(1-P)}{3+v}$ | $\dfrac{vP}{3+v}$ |

Whence:

$$P = \frac{A + \sqrt{(A^2 + 8dn)}}{2n}, \qquad V = \frac{(2+P)(1-P)(3+v)}{4n(v(2+P)+3P)},$$

$$A = a - 2b - 2c - d, \qquad v = \frac{3(c+d)}{a+b}.$$

This estimate of $p$ is independent of $v$ although the variance has terms in $v$.

When the inviability is induced by a dominant gene, the above formula for estimating $P$ can still be used but the variance is different. The variance is now:

$$V = \frac{(2+P)(1-P)(3v+1)}{4n(P(3v+1)+2)}, \qquad v = \frac{a+b}{3(c+d)}.$$

The analysis of the single backcross in conjunction with a recessive inviable gene is very similar to that described earlier. The estimating formula for $p$ does not contain $v$. This indicates that the same formula can be used both for those crosses with a recessive or a dominant debilitating gene. The formula is a cubic:

$$np^3 - (3b + 2c + d)p^2 - (a - 2b + c + 2d)p + 2c = 0.$$

To use this formula for the four possible combinations of linkage phase and whether the $a$ or $b$ locus is assorting in the $3 : 1$ or $1 : 1$ ratio, the following substitution of observed frequencies should be made:

|      | $++$ | $+b$ | $a+$ | $ab$ |
|------|------|------|------|------|
| CIB  | $a$  | $b$  | $c$  | $d$  |
| RIB  | $b$  | $a$  | $d$  | $c$  |
| CBI  | $a$  | $c$  | $b$  | $d$  |
| RBI  | $b$  | $d$  | $a$  | $c$  |

The first row of frequencies in the above tabulation are those given in the formula for $p$. The abbreviations on the left are those employed in Table 5.1. For a dominant gene, substitute $A'$ and $+$ for $+$ and $a$ in the above phenotypes. Solution of the cubic will follow the procedure outlined earlier for perfectly normal assorting genes. The variances will differ, according to the eight situations of Table 5.1. An estimate of $v$ features in the variances and this is given by the formulae in the extreme right column.

The ease by which segregations showing reduced viability and epistasis can be analysed will depend upon the gene affected. If the epistatic gene is inviable, all of the formulae for normal assortment with epistasis can be used since the distinguishable phenotypes will be occurring in the normal ratios. It is only necessary to ensure that the correct situation is chosen.

On the other hand, if one gene is known or suspected to be inviable and the other epistatic, estimation of $p$ and its sampling variance is possible but on a higher level of computational complexity than hitherto encountered. The estimation formulae themselves are not particularly complex but, before the variances can be calculated, an information matrix has to be formed. The variances can then be derived by one of the inversion formulae.

## TABLE 5.1

Expectations and variances in single backcrosses with inviability. Locus $c$ taken as inviable recessive or dominant

| Inviable gene | Locus $a$ $b$ | Phase | Expectations | | | | $V$ | $v$ |
|---|---|---|---|---|---|---|---|---|
| | | | $++$ | $+b$ | $a+$ | $ab$ | | |
| Rec. | I B | C | $\dfrac{2-p}{3+v}$ | $\dfrac{1+p}{3+v}$ | $\dfrac{vp}{3+v}$ | $\dfrac{v(1-p)}{3+v}$ | $\dfrac{3p(1-p)+v(2+p(1-p))(1-p)p}{(3+v)(2-p)(1+p)(1-p)p}$ | $\dfrac{3(c+d)}{a+b}$ |
| Rec. | I B | R | $\dfrac{1+p}{3+v}$ | $\dfrac{2-p}{3+v}$ | $\dfrac{v(1-p)}{3+v}$ | $\dfrac{vp}{3+v}$ | $\dfrac{3p(1-p)+v(2+p(1-p))(1-p)p}{(3+v)(2-p)(1+p)(1-p)p}$ | $\dfrac{3(c+d)}{a+b}$ |
| Rec. | B I | C | $\dfrac{2-p}{2+2v}$ | $\dfrac{p}{2+2v}$ | $\dfrac{v(1+p)}{2+2v}$ | $\dfrac{v(1-p)}{2+2v}$ | $\dfrac{1-p^2+v(2-p)p}{(1+v)(2-p)(1+p)(1-p)p}$ | $\dfrac{c+d}{a+b}$ |
| Rec. | B I | R | $\dfrac{1+p}{2+2v}$ | $\dfrac{1-p}{2+2v}$ | $\dfrac{v(2-p)}{2+2v}$ | $\dfrac{vp}{2+2v}$ | $\dfrac{(2-p)p+v(1-p^2)}{(1+v)(2-p)(1+p)(1-p)p}$ | $\dfrac{c+d}{a+b}$ |
| Dom. | I B | C | $\dfrac{v(2-p)}{1+3v}$ | $\dfrac{v(1+p)}{1+3v}$ | $\dfrac{p}{1+3v}$ | $\dfrac{1-p}{1+3v}$ | $\dfrac{2+(1+3v)p(1-p)}{(1+3v)(2-p)(1+p)(1-p)p}$ | $\dfrac{a+b}{3(c+d)}$ |
| Dom. | I B | R | $\dfrac{v(1+p)}{1+3v}$ | $\dfrac{v(2-p)}{1+3v}$ | $\dfrac{p}{1+3v}$ | $\dfrac{1-p}{1+3v}$ | $\dfrac{2+(1+3v)p(1-p)}{(1+3v)(2-p)(1+p)(1-p)p}$ | $\dfrac{a+b}{3(c+d)}$ |
| Dom. | B I | C | $\dfrac{v(2-p)}{2+2v}$ | $\dfrac{vp}{2+2v}$ | $\dfrac{1+p}{2+2v}$ | $\dfrac{1-p}{2+2v}$ | $\dfrac{(2-p)p+v(1-p^2)}{(1+2v)(2-p)(1+p)(1-p)p}$ | $\dfrac{a+b}{c+d}$ |
| Dom. | B I | R | $\dfrac{v(1+p)}{2+2v}$ | $\dfrac{v(1-p)}{2+2v}$ | $\dfrac{2-p}{2+2v}$ | $\dfrac{p}{2+2v}$ | $\dfrac{(1-p^2)+v(2-p)p}{(1+2v)(1-p)(1+p)(1-p)p}$ | $\dfrac{a+b}{c+d}$ |

Note. Rec. = recessive, Dom. = dominant, I = intercross, B = backcross, C = coupling, R = repulsion.

The simplest situation is that of the testcross. Eight types are possible, depending upon linkage phase, if the epistasis is due to a recessive or dominant gene and if the inviability is due to a recessive or dominant. Taking the case of the coupling testcross in which both the inviable and epistatic genes are recessive as illustrative of the procedure, the expectations are:

|  | ++ | +b | a+, ab |
|---|---|---|---|
| Coupling | $\dfrac{1-p}{1+u}$ | $\dfrac{up}{1+u}$ | $\dfrac{p+u(1-p)}{1+u}$ |
| Observations | $a$ | $b$ | $c$ |

Whence:

$$p = \frac{2b+c \pm \sqrt{(c^2-4ab)}}{2n} \quad \text{and} \quad u = \frac{c \pm \sqrt{(c^2-4ab)}}{2a}.$$

The viability of $b$ is denoted by $u$.

The above formulae do not contain $u$ and it is possible to use it to estimate $p$ for all of the eight cases. By definition, either $a$ or $A'$ will be the recessive or dominant epistatic locus and $b$ or $B'$ will be the recessive or dominant inviable locus. The following substitutions of observed frequencies should be made:

| Phase | Epistasis | Inviability | Substitutions for $p$ | | | Substitutions for $u$ | | |
|---|---|---|---|---|---|---|---|---|
| C | $a$ | $b$ | $a$ | $b$ | $c$ | $a$ | $b$ | $c$ |
| R | $a$ | $b$ | $b$ | $a$ | $c$ | $b$ | $a$ | $c$ |
| C | $a$ | $B'$ | $b$ | $a$ | $c$ | $a$ | $b$ | $c$ |
| R | $a$ | $B'$ | $a$ | $b$ | $c$ | $b$ | $a$ | $c$ |
| C | $A'$ | $b$ | $b$ | $a$ | $c$ | $b$ | $a$ | $c$ |
| R | $A'$ | $b$ | $a$ | $b$ | $c$ | $a$ | $b$ | $c$ |
| C | $A'$ | $B'$ | $a$ | $b$ | $c$ | $b$ | $a$ | $c$ |
| R | $A'$ | $B'$ | $b$ | $a$ | $c$ | $a$ | $b$ | $c$ |

The first row of frequencies in the above tabulation are those given in the formulae for $p$ and $u$. The frequencies for dominant epistasis are found by placing the epistatic class last and taking the distinguishable classes $a+$ and $ab$ as equal to $++$ and $+b$, respectively, for computational purposes.

To derive the exact variance of $p$, it is necessary to calculate an information matrix for $p$ and $u$. This is necessary because these two parameters are not independent (i.e., the $B$ term is not zero). The algebra is tedious but manageable. The three terms of the matrix are shown by Table 5.2. Note that the eight

TABLE 5.2

Formulae for the terms of the information matrix of the testcross with one locus epistatic and one locus inviable

| Phase | Epistasis | Inviability | Matrix terms |
|-------|-----------|-------------|--------------|
| C | $a$ | $b$ | $A = \dfrac{1}{1+u}\left(\dfrac{p+u(1-p)}{(1-p)p} + \dfrac{(1-u)^2}{p+u(1-p)}\right)$ |
| C | $A'$ | $B'$ | $B = \dfrac{1}{(1+u)^2}\left(2 + \dfrac{(1-u)(1-2p)}{p+u(1-p)}\right)$ |
| R | $a$ | $B'$ | |
| R | $A'$ | $b$ | $D = \dfrac{1}{(1+u)^3}\left(\dfrac{p+u(1-p)}{u} + \dfrac{(1-2p)^2}{p+u(1-p)}\right)$ |
| C | $a$ | $B'$ | $A = \dfrac{1}{1+u}\left(\dfrac{1-p(1-u)}{(1-p)p} + \dfrac{(1-u)^2}{1-p(1-u)}\right)$ |
| C | $A'$ | $b$ | $B = \dfrac{1}{(1+u)^2}\left(\dfrac{(1-u)(1-2p)}{1-p(1-u)} - 2\right)$ |
| R | $a$ | $b$ | |
| R | $A'$ | $B'$ | $D = \dfrac{1}{(1+u)^3}\left(\dfrac{1-p(1-u)}{u} + \dfrac{(1-2p)^2}{1-p(1-u)}\right)$ |

cases are divided into two groups, each with slightly different formulae for the terms of the matrix. The variance is then:

$$V = \frac{D}{n(Ad - B^2)}.$$

Intercrosses with epistatic and inviable loci can be analysed in a similar manner. As usual for this type of cross, estimation will be for $P$ in the first instance. Four situations have to be considered, depending whether the epistasis is due to a recessive or dominant gene and likewise for the inviability. Two formulae are necessary to estimate $P$ and four to estimate $u$ as shown by Table 5.3. By definition, the observed frequencies will be symbolized as:

|  | $++$ | $+b$ | $a+$, $ab$ |
|---|---|---|---|
| Recessive epistasis | $a$ | $b$ | $c$ |

|  | $++$ | $+b$ | $A'+$, $A'b$ |
|---|---|---|---|
| Dominant epistasis | $a$ | $b$ | $c$ |

TABLE 5.3

Estimation of the crossover fraction and viability for the intercross with one locus epistatic and one locus inviable

---

$a$ epistatic, $b$ inviable

$$P = \frac{2a - 2b - c - \sqrt{[(2b+3c)^2 - 12ab]}}{2n}$$

$$u = \frac{2b + 3c - \sqrt{[2b+3c]^2 - 12ab]}}{2a}$$

$a$ epistatic, $B$ inviable

$P$ = as above.

$$u = \frac{2b + 3c - \sqrt{[(2b+3c)^2 - 12ab]}}{6b}$$

$A'$ epistatic, $b$ inviable

$$P = \frac{a - 2b + 2c - \sqrt{[(a-2b)^2 - 12bc]}}{2b}$$

$$u = \frac{a - 2b - \sqrt{[(a-2b)^2 - 12ab]}}{2b}$$

$A'$ epistatic, $B$ inviable

$P$ = as above.

$$u = \frac{a - 2b - \sqrt{[(a-2b)^2 - 12ab]}}{6c}$$

---

TABLE 5.4

Formulae for the terms of the information matrices of the intercross, with
one locus epistatic and one locus inviable

---

$a$ epistatic, $b$ inviable

$$A = \frac{1}{3+u}\left(\frac{1-P+u(2+P)}{(2+P)(1-P)} + \frac{(1-u)^2}{1-P(1-u)}\right)$$

$$B = \frac{1}{(3+u)^2}\left(\frac{(1-u)(1-4P)}{1-P(1-u)} - 4\right)$$

$$D = \frac{1}{(3+u)^3}\left(\frac{9(1-P)+u(2+P)}{u} + \frac{(1-4P)^2}{1-P(1-u)}\right)$$

$a$ epistatic, $B'$ inviable

$$A = \frac{1}{3u+1}\left(\frac{2+P+u(1-P)}{(2+P)(1-P)} + \frac{(1-u)^2}{P+u(1-P)}\right)$$

$$B = \frac{1}{3u+1}\left(4 - \frac{(1-u)(1-4P)}{P+u(1-P)}\right)$$

$$D = \frac{1}{3u+1}\left(\frac{2+P+9u(1-P)}{u} + \frac{(1-4P)^2}{P+u(1-P)}\right)$$

$A'$ epistatic, $b$ inviable

$$A = \frac{1}{3+u}\left(\frac{P+u(1-P)}{(1-P)P} + \frac{(1-u)^2}{2+P+u(1-P)}\right)$$

$$B = \frac{1}{(3+u)^2}\left(4 + \frac{(1-u)(1-4P)}{2+P+u(1-P)}\right)$$

$$D = \frac{1}{(3+u)^3}\left(\frac{9P+u(1-P)}{u} + \frac{(1-4P)^2}{2+P+u(1-P)}\right)$$

$A'$ epistatic, $B'$ inviable

$$A = \frac{1}{3u+1}\left(\frac{1-P(1-u)}{(1-P)P} + \frac{(1-u)^2}{1-P+u(2+P)}\right)$$

$$B = \frac{1}{(3u+1)^2}\left(\frac{(1-u)(1-4P)}{1-P+u(2+P)} - 4\right)$$

$$D = \frac{1}{(3u+1)^3}\left(\frac{1-P+9uP}{u} - \frac{(1-4P)^2}{1-P+u(2+P)}\right)$$

---

Table 5.4 gives formulae for the terms of the information matrix for each of the four possible situations. The variance is then:

$$V = \frac{D}{4nP(AD - B^2)}.$$

The single backcross with epistatic and inviability can be dealt with similarly. There are sixteen different situations arising from the combination of linkage phase, whether the epistatic or inviable genes are recessive or dominant, respectively, and are assorting in a 1 : 1 or 3 : 1 ratio. The estimating formulae for $p$ and $u$ are given in Table 5.5. The observed frequencies $a$, $b$, and $c$ represent the same phenotype

TABLE 5.5

Estimation of the crossover fraction and viability for the single backcross with one locus epistatic and one locus inviable

---

CIB, $a$ epistatic, $b$ inviable

$$p = \frac{3b + c - a - \sqrt{[(n + 2c)^2 - 16ab]}}{2n}$$

$$u = \frac{n + 2c - \sqrt{[(n + 2c)^2 - 16ab]}}{4a}$$

RIB, $a$ epistatic, $b$ inviable

$$p = \frac{3a - c - b - \sqrt{[(n + c)^2 - 16ab]}}{2n}$$

$u$ = as above

CBI, $a$ epistatic, $b$ inviable

$$p = \frac{3b + 2c - a - \sqrt{[(b + 2c - a)^2 - 12ab]}}{2n}$$

$$u = \frac{b + 2c - a - \sqrt{[(b + 2c - a)^2 - 12ab]}}{2a}$$

RBI, $a$ epistatic, $b$ inviable

$$p = \frac{3a - b - \sqrt{[(b + 2c - a)^2 - 12ab]}}{2n}$$

$u$ = as above

Table 5.5—*cont.*

CIB, $a$ epistatic, $B'$ inviable

$$p = \frac{3b+c-a-\sqrt{[(n+2c)^2-16ab]}}{2n}$$

$$u = \frac{n+2c-\sqrt{[(n+2c)^2-16ab]}}{4b}$$

RIB, $a$ epistatic, $B'$ inviable

$$p = \frac{3a+c-b-\sqrt{[(n+2c)^2-16ab]}}{2n}$$

$$u = \frac{n+2c-\sqrt{[(n+2c)^2-16ab]}}{4a}$$

CBI, $a$ epistatic, $B'$ inviable

$$p = \frac{3b+2c-a-\sqrt{[(b+2c-a)^2-12ab]}}{2n}$$

$$u = \frac{b+2c-a-\sqrt{[(b+2c-a)^2-12ab]}}{6b}$$

RBI, $a$ epistatic, $B'$ inviable

$$p = \frac{3a-b-\sqrt{[(b+2c-a)^2-12ab]}}{2n}$$

$$u = \frac{n+2c-a-\sqrt{[(b+2c-a)^2-12ab]}}{6b}$$

CIB, $A'$ epistatic, $b$ inviable

$$p = \frac{3a+c-b-\sqrt{[(c-a-b)^2-16ab]}}{2n}$$

$$u = \frac{c-a-b-\sqrt{[(c-a-b)^2-16ab]}}{4a}$$

RIB, $A'$ epistatic, $b$ inviable

$$p = \frac{3b+c-b-\sqrt{[(c-a-b)^2-12ab]}}{2n}$$

$$u = \frac{c-a-b-\sqrt{[(c-a-b)^2-12ab]}}{4a}$$

CBI, $A'$ epistatic, $b$ inviable

$$p = \frac{3a-b-\sqrt{[(b+2c-a)^2-12ab]}}{2n}$$

$$u = \frac{b+2c-a-\sqrt{[(b+2c-a)^2-12ab]}}{2a}$$

Table 5.5—*cont.*

RBI, $A'$ epistatic, $b$ inviable

$$p = \frac{3b+2c-a-\sqrt{[(b+2c-a)^2-12ab]}}{2n}$$

$$u = \frac{b+2c-a-\sqrt{[(b+2c-a)^2-12ab]}}{2a}$$

CBI, $A'$ epistatic, $B'$ inviable

$$p = \frac{3a+c-b-\sqrt{[(c-a-b)^2-16ab]}}{2n}$$

$$u = \frac{c-a-b-\sqrt{[(c-a-b)^2-16ab]}}{4b}$$

RIB, $A'$ epistatic, $B'$ inviable

$$p = \frac{3b+c-a-\sqrt{[(c-a-b)^2-12ab]}}{2n}$$

$$u = \frac{c-a-b-\sqrt{[(c-a-b)^2-12ab]}}{4b}$$

CBI, $A'$ epistatic, $B'$ inviable

$$p = \frac{3a-b-\sqrt{[(b+2c-a)^2-12ab]}}{2n}$$

$$u = \frac{b+2c-a-\sqrt{[(b+2c-a)^2-12ab]}}{6b}$$

RBI, $A'$ epistatic, $B'$ inviable

$$p = \frac{3b+2c-a-\sqrt{[(b+2c-a)^2-12ab]}}{2n}$$

$$u = \frac{b+2c-a-\sqrt{[(b+2c-a)^2-12ab]}}{6b}$$

Note: C = coupling, R = repulsion, B = backcross, I = intercross.

classes as for the intercross. Table 5.6 gives formulae for the terms of the appropriate matrix. The precise term for any segregation is found by substitution in the general formulae. The two columns on the left side are the segregations; the first gives the mating type and the second, the genes showing epistasis and inviability, respectively. The variance is then:

$$V = \frac{D}{n(AD-B^2)}.$$

TABLE 5.6

Formulae for the terms of the information matrices of the single backcross
with one locus epistatic and one locus inviable

$$A = \frac{1}{A}\left(\frac{B+uC}{BC} + \frac{(1-u)^2}{G}\right)$$

$$B = \frac{1}{A^2}\left(D + \frac{2(1-u)(1-2p)}{G}\right)$$

$$D = \frac{1}{A^3}\left(\frac{E+F}{u} + \frac{4(1-2p)^2}{G}\right)$$

Substitute in the above as follows:

|  |  | $A$ | $B$ | $C$ | $D$ | $E$ | $F$ | $G$ |
|---|---|---|---|---|---|---|---|---|
| CIB | $ab$ | $2(1+u)$ | $1+p$ | $2-p$ | $4$ | $4(1+p)$ | $4(2-p)$ | $p+u(1-p)$ |
| RIB | $ab$ | $2(1+u)$ | $2-p$ | $1+p$ | $-4$ | $4(2-p)$ | $4(1+p)$ | $1-p(1-u)$ |
| CBI | $ab$ | $3+u$ | $p$ | $2-p$ | $4$ | $9p$ | $2-p$ | $1+p+u(1-p)$ |
| RBI | $ab$ | $1+u$ | $1-p$ | $1+p$ | $-4$ | $9(1-p)$ | $1+u$ | $2-p(1-u)$ |
| CIB | $aB'$ | $2(1+u)$ | $2-p$ | $1+p$ | $-4$ | $4(2-p)$ | $4(1+u)$ | $1-p(1-u)$ |
| RIB | $aB'$ | $2(1+u)$ | $1+p$ | $2-p$ | $4$ | $4(1+p)$ | $4(2-p)$ | $p+u(1-p)$ |
| CBI | $aB'$ | $3u+1$ | $2-p$ | $p$ | $-4$ | $2-p$ | $9p$ | $1-p+u(1+p)$ |
| RBI | $aB'$ | $3u+1$ | $1+p$ | $1-p$ | $4$ | $1+p$ | $9(1-p)$ | $p+u(2-p)$ |
| CIB | $A'b$ | $2(1+u)$ | $1-p$ | $p$ | $-4$ | $4(1-p)$ | $4p$ | $2-p+u(1+p)$ |
| RIB | $A'b$ | $2(1+u)$ | $p$ | $1-p$ | $4$ | $4p$ | $4(1-p)$ | $1+p+u(2-p)$ |
| CBI | $A'b$ | $3+u$ | $1-p$ | $1+p$ | $-4$ | $1-p$ | $9(1+p)$ | $2-p(1-u)$ |
| RBI | $A'b$ | $3+u$ | $p$ | $2-p$ | $4$ | $p$ | $9(2-p)$ | $1+p+u(1-p)$ |
| CIB | $A'B'$ | $2(1+u)$ | $1-p$ | $p$ | $4$ | $4p$ | $4(1-p)$ | $1+p+u(2-p)$ |
| RIB | $A'B'$ | $2(1+u)$ | $1-p$ | $p$ | $-4$ | $4(1-p)$ | $4p$ | $2-p+u(1+p)$ |
| CBI | $A'B'$ | $3u+1$ | $1+p$ | $1-p$ | $4$ | $9(1+p)$ | $1-p$ | $p+u(2-p)$ |
| RBI | $A'B'$ | $3u+1$ | $2-p$ | $p$ | $-4$ | $9(2-p)$ | $p$ | $1-p+u(1-p)$ |

Note: The second column indicates the epistatic and inviable gene, respectively,
corresponding to the entries of the preceding table.

### Two Inviable Loci

A problem with experiments involving two semi-viable genes is whether these may interact with each other to reduce the frequency below that expected if each were acting alone. However, if it can be assumed that there is no interaction or that the interaction is trivial, then consistent estimates of the crossover value can be found without too much difficulty. In previous sections, the $a$ locus has been represented as possessing the partially inviable allele and symbolized as $v$. The inviability of the $b$ locus may conveniently be symbolized as $u$.

The testcross still ranks as an efficienct method of investigation provided individuals homozygous for the two inviable genes are able to reproduce. The expectations are:

|  | $++$ | $+b$ | $a+$ | $ab$ |
|---|---|---|---|---|
| Coupling | $\dfrac{1-p}{D}$ | $\dfrac{up}{D}$ | $\dfrac{vp}{D}$ | $\dfrac{uv(1-p)}{D}$ |
| Repulsion | $\dfrac{p}{D}$ | $\dfrac{u(1-p)}{D}$ | $\dfrac{v(1-p)}{D}$ | $\dfrac{uvp}{D}$ |

Where, $D = (1+vu)(1-p)+(u+v)p$ for coupling and $D = (1+vu)p+(u+v)(1-p)$ for repulsion. Whence:

Coupling
$$p = \frac{\sqrt{bc}}{\sqrt{ad}+\sqrt{bc}}.$$

Repulsion
$$p = \frac{\sqrt{ad}}{\sqrt{ad}+\sqrt{bc}}.$$

also
$$v = \sqrt{\frac{cd}{ab}}, \qquad u = \sqrt{\frac{bd}{ac}}.$$

The above formulae are for the common situation of two recessive inviable genes. The similar situations of two dominant genes or one recessive and one dominant gene can be analysed by interchanging the appropriate class phenotypes. Formulae for the terms of the relevant matrix are given in Table 5.7. The variance is then:

$$V = \frac{DF - E^2}{n[A(DF - E^2) + B(2CE - BF) - C^2 D]}$$

TABLE 5.7

Formulae for the terms of the information matrices of the testcross with two inviable genes

| Term | Coupling | Repulsion |
|------|----------|-----------|
| A | $\dfrac{AB[B - p(A + B)]}{p(1-p)D^3}$ | $\dfrac{AB[A - p(A + B)]}{p(1-p)D^3}$ |
| B | $\dfrac{(1 - u^2)(vC \mid E)}{D^3}$ | $\dfrac{(u^2 - 1)(C + vE)}{D^3}$ |
| C | $\dfrac{(1 - v^2)(uF + G)}{D^3}$ | $\dfrac{(v^2 - 1)(F + uG)}{D^3}$ |
| D | $\dfrac{CE(vC + E)}{vD^3}$ | $\dfrac{CE(C + vE)}{vD^3}$ |
| E | $\dfrac{(1 - 2p)(vC + E)}{D^3}$ | $\dfrac{(1 - 2p)(C + vE)}{D^3}$ |
| F | $\dfrac{FG(uF + G)}{uD^3}$ | $\dfrac{FG(F + uG)}{uD^3}$ |

Where: $A = u + v$, $B = 1 + uv$, $C = p + u(1 - p)$,

$E = 1 - u(1 - p)$, $F = p + v(1 - p)$, $G = 1 - v(1 - p)$;

and $D = pA + (1 - p)B$ for coupling and $(1 - p)A + pB$ for repulsion.

Bailey (1949b) has derived the following approximation for the variance of the testcross which is satisfactory for most purposes:

$$V = \frac{p^2(1 - p)^2[(a + b)cd + (c + d)ab]}{4(abcd)}.$$

When data are available for both linkage phases, an elegant analysis may be used (Fisher, 1951). This makes explicit use of the principle that balancing the phases tends to cancel inviability effects. The observed frequencies are written as:

Phenotypes

|  | $++, ab$ | $+b, a+$ |
|---|---|---|
| Coupling | $a$ | $b$ |
| Repulsion | $c$ | $d$ |

Whence:

$$p = \frac{\sqrt{bc}}{\sqrt{ad} + \sqrt{bc}}$$

and

$$V = \frac{p^2(1-p)^2[(a+b)cd + (c+d)ab]}{4abcd}.$$

These formulae are identical to those given earlier but note that the class frequencies are quite different. The amount of arithmetic is reduced but estimation of the viabilities for each gene cannot be obtained. Fisher has discussed how the variance can be minimized as the experiment proceeds by ensuring that the two products $ab$ and $cd$ are kept approximately numerically equal by adjusting the total number of coupling and repulsion offspring.

The intercross gives rise to three situations, depending upon whether one or both of the semi-viable genes are recessive or dominant. The expectations are:

|  | $++$ | $+b$ | $a+$ | $ab$ |
|---|---|---|---|---|
| Two recessive inviable genes | $\dfrac{2+P}{D}$ | $\dfrac{u(1-p)}{D}$ | $\dfrac{v(1-p)}{D}$ | $\dfrac{uvP}{D}$ |
|  | $A'B'$ | $A'+$ | $+B'$ | $++$ |
| Two dominant inviable genes | $\dfrac{uv(2+P)}{D}$ | $\dfrac{v(1-P)}{D}$ | $\dfrac{u(1-P)}{D}$ | $\dfrac{P}{D}$ |
|  | $A'+$ | $A'b$ | $++$ | $+b$ |
| Genes $A'$ and $b$ inviable | $\dfrac{v(2+P)}{D}$ | $\dfrac{uv(1-P)}{D}$ | $\dfrac{1-P}{D}$ | $\dfrac{uP}{D}$ |

Where $D$ is given by the respective Table 5.8, 5.9, or 5.10. The formula for $P$ is the same for each but those for $v$ and $u$ will differ. The estimator for $P$ is:

$$P = \frac{ad+bc-\sqrt{[bc(3ad+bc)]}}{ad-bc}.$$

For two recessive inviable genes:

$$v = \frac{bc+\sqrt{[bc(3ad+bc)]}}{ab},$$

$$u = \frac{bc+\sqrt{[bc(3ad+bc)]}}{ac} = \frac{bv}{c}.$$

For two dominant inviable genes:

$$v = \frac{\sqrt{[bc(3ad+bc)]}-bc}{3cd},$$

$$u = \frac{\sqrt{[bc(3ad+bc)]}-bc}{3bd} = \frac{cv}{b}.$$

For $A'$ and $b$ inviable genes:

$$v = \frac{\sqrt{[bc(3ad+bc)]}-bc}{3cd},$$

$$u = \frac{bc+\sqrt{[bc(3ad+bc)]}}{ac} = \frac{3dv}{a}.$$

The variance of $p$ can be derived from the matrix elements of tables 5.8, 5.9, and 5.10, according to the nature of the intercross. The variance is then:

$$V = \frac{DF-E^2}{4nP[A(DF-E^2)+B(2CE-BF)-C^2D]}.$$

The single backcross tends to be useful in present circumstances, especially if the double inviable class is infertile or too weak for successful reproduction. There are eight possible situations depending on phase and whether one or both of the inviable genes are recessive or dominant. In each situation, locus $a$ is defined as segregating in the 3 : 1 ratio. The formulae for $p$, $v$, and $u$ are different in each instance except that the four cases in which one inviable gene is recessive and the other dominant duplicate one or the other of the cases in which both genes are either recessive or dominant.

TABLE 5.8

Formulae for the terms of the information matrix of the intercross with two inviable recessive genes

$$A = \frac{1}{D^3}\left(\frac{A^2}{2+P} + \frac{(u+v)B^2}{1-P} + \frac{uvC^2}{P}\right)$$

$$B = \frac{1}{D^3}\,[(u+1)^2 - 4]\,(vE+F)$$

$$C = \frac{1}{D^3}\,[(v+1)^2 - 4]\,(uG+H)$$

$$D = \frac{EF}{vD^3}\,(vE+F)$$

$$E = \frac{1}{D^3}\,(4P-1)(vE+F)$$

$$F = \frac{GH}{uD^3}\,(uG+H)$$

Where: $A = 3(u+v)-2uv$, $B = 3+uv$, $C = 2+u+v$,

$D = 2+P+(u+v)(1-P)+uvP$, $E = 1-u(1-P)$

$F = 2+P+u(1-P)$, $G = 1-P(1-v)$, $H = 2+P+v(1-P)$.

---

TABLE 5.9

Formulae for the terms of the information matrix for the intercross with two inviable dominant genes

$$A = \frac{1}{D^3}\left(\frac{uvA^2}{2+P} + \frac{(u+v)B^2}{1-P} + \frac{C^2}{P}\right)$$

$$B = \frac{1}{D^3}\,[4v^2 - (1+v)^2]\,(E+uF)$$

$$C = \frac{1}{D^3}\,[4v^2 - (1+v)^2]\,(E+uF)$$

$$D = \frac{EF}{vD^3}\,(E+vF)$$

$$E = \frac{1}{D^3}\,(4P-1)(E+vF)$$

$$F = \frac{GH}{uD^3}\,(G+vH)$$

Where: $A = 3(u+v)-2$, $B = 1+3uv$, $C = 2uv+u+v$,

$D = uv(2+P)+(u+v)(1-P)+P$, $E = P+u(1-P)$,

$F = 1-P+u(2+P)$, $G = P+v(1-P)$, $H = 1-P+v(2+P)$.

TABLE 5.10 87

Formulae for the terms of the information matrix for the intercross with
one dominant $(A')$ and one recessive $(b)$ inviable gene

$$A = \frac{1}{D^3}\left(\frac{vA^2}{2+P} + \frac{(1+uv)B^2}{1-P} + \frac{uC^2}{P}\right)$$

$$B = \frac{1}{D^3}[4-(1-u)^2](E+vF)$$

$$C = \frac{1}{D^3}[(1+v)^2-4v^2](uG+H)$$

$$D = \frac{EF}{vD^3}(E+vF)$$

$$E = \frac{1}{D^3}(1-4P)(E+vF)$$

$$F = \frac{GH}{uD^3}(uG+H)$$

Where: $A = 3-2u+3uv$, $B = 3v+u$, $C = 1+v(2+u)$,

$D = 1+v(2+P)-(1-u)P+uv(1-P)$, $E = 1-P(1-u)$,

$F = 2+P+u(1-P)$, $G = P+v(1-P)$, $H = 1-P+v(2+P)$.

The duplication depends upon linkage phase and whether the dominant gene is $A'$ or $B'$. When $A'$ is the affected gene, the coupling or repulsion case is identical to that for repulsion or coupling, respectively, where both dominant genes are affected. It is merely necessary to substitute the frequencies $b$, $a$, $d$, and $c$ of the former for the phenotypic class frequencies $a$, $b$, $c$, and $d$, respectively, of the latter. Similarly, when $B'$ is the affected gene, the coupling or repulsion case is identical to that for repulsion or coupling, respectively, where both recessive genes are affected. It is merely necessary to substitute the frequencies $b$, $a$, $d$, and $c$ of the former for the class frequencies $a$, $b$, $c$, and $d$, respectively, of the latter. The appropriate formulae of Tables 5.11, 5.12, 5.13, 5.14, and 5.15 can then be employed.

The variance of $p$ can be derived from the matrix elements shown in Tables 5.12, 5.13, 5.14, and 5.15, according to the nature of the single backcross. The variance is then

$$V = \frac{DF-E^2}{n[A(DF-E^2)+B(2CE-BF)-C^2D]}.$$

TABLE 5.11

Estimation of the crossover function and viabilities for the single backcross
with two inviable genes

---

CIB, $a$ and $b$ inviable

$$p = \frac{3bc + ad - \sqrt{[(ad + bc)^2 + 12abcd]}}{2(bc - ad)}$$

$$v = \frac{ad + bc + \sqrt{[(ad + bc)^2 + 12abcd]}}{2ab}$$

$$u = \frac{ad + bc + \sqrt{[(ad + bc)^2 + 12abcd]}}{4ac}$$

RIB, $a$ and $b$ inviable

$$p = \frac{3ad + bc - \sqrt{[(ad + bc)^2 + 12abcd]}}{2(ad - bc)}$$

$v$ = same as $v$ above

$u$ = same as $u$ above

CIB, $A'$ and $B'$ inviable

$$p = \frac{3bc + ad - \sqrt{[(ad + bc)^2 + 12abcd]}}{2(bc - ad)}$$

$$u = \frac{\sqrt{[(ad + bc)^2 + 12abcd]} - (ad + bc)}{6cd}$$

$$v = \frac{ad + bc + \sqrt{[(ad + bc)^2 + 12abcd]}}{4bd}$$

RIB, $A'$ and $B'$ inviable

$$p = \frac{3ad + bc - \sqrt{[(ad + bc)^2 + 12abcd]}}{2(ad - bc)}$$

$v$ = same as $v$ above

$u$ = same as $u$ above

---

Many of the calculations for the variance may seem tedious
at first blush but this is the price exacted for precise treatment.
Fortunately, the calculations are tedious, rather than difficult,
and the tedium can be alleviated by machine computation.
Alternatively, by the aid of maximum likelihood scores, it is

TABLE 5.12

Formulae for the terms of the information matrix for the coupling single backcross with two inviable recessive genes

$$A = \frac{1}{D^3}\left(\frac{A^2}{2-p} + \frac{uB^2}{1+p} + \frac{vC^2}{p} + \frac{uvE^2}{1-p}\right)$$

$$B = \frac{2}{D^3}(1-u^2)(vF+G)$$

$$C = \frac{1}{D^3}[4-(1+u)^2](uH+J)$$

$$D = \frac{FG}{vD^3}(vF+G)$$

$$E = \frac{2}{D^3}(1-2p)(vF+G)$$

$$F = \frac{HJ}{uD^3}(uH+J)$$

Where: $A = 3u+v(2-u)$, $B = 3-v(1-2u)$, $C = 2+u(1+v)$,

$D = 2-p+u(1+p)+vp+uv(1-p)$, $E = 1+2u+v$, $F = p+u(1-p)$,

$G = 2-p+u(1+p)$, $H = 1+p+v(1-p)$, $J = 2-p(1-v)$.

possible to make use of the approximate formula for the realized information:

$$V_p = \frac{p_1-p_2}{Sp_1-Sp_2},$$

where scores have been computed for two sufficiently close values of $p$ of opposite sign (sufficiently close meaning a difference of not more than one per cent). This approximation seems attractive but the calculation of two sets of scores can involve lengthy arithmetic and algebra, too, if the scores are not already to hand for the particular cross.

In general, it would seen politic to avoid experiments with two inviable loci unless the rewards warrant the extra time and effort which are often demanded. There is a statistical aspect, moreover, which is of importance. Unless a four class segregation can be fully recorded, there will be insufficient

GMLM-4

## TABLE 5.13

Formulae for the terms of the information matrix for the repulsion single backcross with two inviable recessive genes

$$A = \frac{1}{D^3}\left(\frac{A^2}{1+p} + \frac{uB^2}{2-p} + \frac{vC^2}{1-p} + \frac{uvD^2}{p}\right)$$

$$B = \frac{2}{D^3}(u^2-1)(vF+G)$$

$$C = \frac{1}{D^3}[(1+v)^2-4](uH+J)$$

$$D = \frac{FG}{vD^3}(F+vG)$$

$$E = \frac{2}{D^3}(2p-1)(vF+G)$$

$$F = \frac{HJ}{uD^3}(H+uJ)$$

Where: $A = 3u+v(2-u)$, $B = 3-v(1-2u)$, $C = 2+u(1+v)$,
$D = 1+p+u(2-p)+v(1-p)+uvp$, $E = 1+2u+v$, $F = 1-p(1-u)$,
$G = 1+p+u(2-p)$, $H = 2-p(1-v)$, $J = 1+p+v(1-p)$.

## TABLE 5.14

Formulae for the terms of the information matrix for the coupling single backcross with two inviable dominant genes

$$A = \frac{1}{D^3}\left(\frac{uvA^2}{2-p} + \frac{vB^2}{1+p} + \frac{uC^2}{p} + \frac{E^2}{1-p}\right)$$

$$B = \frac{2}{D^3}(1-u^2)(F+vG)$$

$$C = \frac{1}{D^3}[(1+v)^2-4v^2](H+uJ)$$

$$D = \frac{FG}{D^3}(vF+G)$$

$$E = \frac{2}{D^3}(1-2p)(F+vG)$$

$$F = \frac{HJ}{uD^3}(uH+J)$$

Where: $A = 3v+2u-1$, $B = 2-u(1-3v)$, $C = 1+v(1+2u)$,
$D = 1-p(1-u)+v(1+p)+uv(2-p)$, $E = 2v+u(1+v)$,
$F = 1-p(1-u)$, $G = 1+p+u(2-p)$, $H = 1-p+v(1+p)$,
$J = p+v(2-p)$.

## TABLE 5.15

Formulae for the terms of the information matrix for the repulsion single backcross with two inviable dominant genes

$$A = \frac{1}{D^3}\left(\frac{uvA^2}{1+p} + \frac{vB^2}{2-p} + \frac{uC^2}{1-p} + \frac{E^2}{p}\right)$$

$$B = \frac{2}{D^3}(u^2-1)(F+vG)$$

$$C = \frac{1}{D^3}[Gv^2-(1+v)^2](H+uJ)$$

$$D = \frac{FG}{vD^3}(F+vG)$$

$$E = \frac{2}{D^3}(2p-1)(F+vG)$$

$$F = \frac{HJ}{uD^3}(H+uJ)$$

Where: $A = 3v+2u-1$, $B = 2-u(1-3v)$, $C = 1+v(1+2u)$,

$D = p+u(1-p)+v(2-p)+uv(1+p)$, $E = 2v+u(1+v)$,

$F = p+u(1-p)$, $G = 2-p+u(1+p)$, $H = p+v(2-p)$,

$J = 1-p+v(1+p)$.

degrees of freedom to permit estimation of all of the relevant parameters. For example, estimation of the crossover fraction would be impossible, should epistasis also be involved, unless it is feasible to employ estimates of the viability gained from other experiments. The balancing of linkage phases is the practical approach for most cases which have to be investigated. It should not be imagined that this approach will solve all problems but it is powerful enough to yield useful results.

# CHAPTER 6

# Estimation with Impenetrance

Impenetrance may not be of such frequent occurrence as inviability but it is frequent enough to warrant consideration. In common with inviability, a small departure from normal assortment due to impenetrance may not have much effect, whereas a large departure cannot be lightly ignored, since it will almost certainly produce misleading estimates of the crossover value. This chapter deals with the formulae to be employed for many of the more common situations involving one or two loci with impenetrant alleles. Relevant papers on estimation with impenetrance are Bailey (1950), Sanchez-Monge (1962), and Allard and Adler (1960).

## ONE IMPENETRANT LOCUS

The simplest situation is that of the testcross involving a single impenetrant gene. Locus $a$ will be taken as having the impenetrant gene. Four possibilities may occur, depending upon linkage phase and whether the impenetrance is due to a recessive or dominant gene. The expectations for the coupling testcross with impenetrance of a recessive gene are:

| $++$ | $+b$ | $a+$ | $ab$ |
|------|------|------|------|
| $\dfrac{1-\alpha p}{2}$ | $\dfrac{1-\alpha(1-p)}{2}$ | $\dfrac{\alpha p}{2}$ | $\dfrac{\alpha(1-p)}{2}$ |

| Observations | $a$ | $b$ | $c$ | $d$ |
|---|---|---|---|---|

Whence:

$$p = \frac{c(b+d)}{d(a+c)+c(b+d)}, \qquad \alpha = \frac{d(a+c)+c(b+d)}{(a+c)(b+d)}.$$

The symmetrical nature of the expectations for the testcross enables the above formulae to be used for all four situations. It is merely necessary to interchange the phenotype class frequencies as indicated in the following:

| Impenetrant gene | Phase | Frequencies | | | |
|---|---|---|---|---|---|
| $a$ | Coupling | $a$ | $b$ | $c$ | $d$ |
| $a$ | Repulsion | $b$ | $a$ | $d$ | $c$ |
| $A'$ | Coupling | $c$ | $d$ | $a$ | $b$ |
| $A'$ | Repulsion | $d$ | $c$ | $b$ | $a$ |

Unlike the simpler situations with inviability, it is not possible to obtain variance estimates independent of $\alpha$. This means that terms of a matrix have to be calculated in the first instance and formulae for these are given in Table 6.1. The variance is then:

$$V = \frac{D}{n(AD - B^2)}.$$

Bailey (1950) has derived the following approximation for the variance of the testcross:

$$V = \frac{2(1-p)p[1 - 2\alpha(1-p)p]}{\alpha n}.$$

The intercross will give rise to two situations, depending whether the impenetrant gene is recessive or dominant. In each

TABLE 6.1

Formulae for the terms of the information matrix of the testcross with one gene impenetrant

$$A = \frac{\alpha[1 - \alpha + 2\alpha p(1-p)]}{2(1-p)p[1 - \alpha(1-p)](1 - \alpha p)}$$

$$B = \frac{\alpha(2p - 1)}{2[1 - \alpha(1-p)](1 - \alpha p)}$$

$$C = \frac{1 - 2\alpha p(1-p)}{2\alpha[1 - \alpha(1-p)](1 - \alpha p)}$$

case, the initial estimate is of $P$, from which $p$ is derived by one of the usual relations. The expectations for the intercross involving a recessive gene are:

| $++$ | $+b$ | $a+$ | $ab$ |
|------|------|------|------|
| $\dfrac{3-\alpha(1-P)}{4}$ | $\dfrac{1-\alpha P}{4}$ | $\dfrac{\alpha(1-P)}{4}$ | $\dfrac{\alpha P}{4}$ |

Whence:

$$P=\frac{d(a+c)}{d(a+c)+3c(b+d)}, \qquad \alpha=\frac{d(a+c)+3c(b+d)}{(a+c)(b+d)}.$$

The expectations for the intercross involving a dominant impenetrant gene are:

| $A'+$ | $A'b$ | $++$ | $+b$ |
|-------|-------|------|------|
| $\dfrac{\alpha(2+P)}{4}$ | $\dfrac{\alpha(1-P)}{4}$ | $\dfrac{3-\alpha(2+P)}{4}$ | $\dfrac{1-\alpha(1-P)}{4}$ |

Whence:

$$P=\frac{a(b+3d)-2bc}{b(a+c)+3a(b+d)}, \qquad \alpha=\frac{b(a+c)+3a(b+d)}{3(a+c)(b+d)}.$$

As before, matrix elements have to be calculated before an exact estimation of the variance can be obtained. These are shown in Table 6.2 and 6.3, respectively. The variance is then:

$$V=\frac{D}{4nP(AD-B^2)}.$$

TABLE 6.2

Formulae for the terms of the information matrix of the intercross with a recessive impenetrant gene

$$A=\frac{\alpha[3-\alpha+2\alpha P(1-2P)]}{4(1-P)P[3-\alpha(1-P)](1-\alpha P)}$$

$$B=\frac{\alpha(4P-1)}{[3-\alpha(1-P)](1-\alpha P)}$$

$$D=\frac{3-4\alpha P(1-P)}{4\alpha[3-\alpha(1-P)](1-\alpha P)}$$

TABLE 6.3

Formulae for the terms of the information matrix of the intercross with a
dominant impenetrant gene

$$A = \frac{\alpha[9-7\alpha+2\alpha P(1-2P)]}{4(2+P)(1-P)[3-\alpha(2+P)][1-\alpha(1-P)]}$$

$$B = \frac{\alpha(4P-1)}{4[3-\alpha(2+P)][1-\alpha(1-P)]}$$

$$D = \frac{9-8\alpha+4\alpha P(1+P)}{4\alpha[3-\alpha(2+P)][1-\alpha(1-P)]}$$

The single backcross presents a number of situations. There
are eight possibilities, depending upon phase, whether the
backcrossed or intercrossed gene is showing impenetrance and
whether it is a recessive or dominant gene. Not all of these are
different, however. Four of the possibilities duplicate the other
four after suitable interchange of classes so that the designated
frequencies have identical expectations. Table 6.4 gives
formulae for the distinguishable cases. The table also shows the
appropriate substitutions of frequencies for the other four
situations.

The matrix elements for the various crosses are shown by
Table 6.5. Only the four distinguishable cases are listed, the
other four will have the same elements as the cross which they
duplicate. The variance is then:

$$V = \frac{D}{n(AD-B^2)}.$$

The problems presented by segregations showing impenetrance and epistatis can be tackled by extension of the above
methods. If the epistatic gene itself shows impenetrance, the
series of formulae are similar to those given previously but, if
anything, slightly simpler. Taking the coupling testcross with a
recessive gene as illustrative and defining locus $a$ as both
epistatic and impenetrant, the expectations are:

|  | $++$ | $+b$ | $a+, ab$ |
|---|---|---|---|
| Expectations | $\dfrac{1-\alpha p}{2}$ | $\dfrac{1-\alpha(1-p)}{2}$ | $\dfrac{\alpha}{2}$ |

Observations                   $a$                        $b$                        $c$

Whence:

$$p = \frac{b+c-a}{2c}, \qquad \alpha = \frac{2c}{n}.$$

TABLE 6.4

Estimation of the crossover fraction and penetrance for the single backcross

---

CIB, $a$ impenetrant

$$p = \frac{c(b+d)}{d(a+c)+c(b+d)}$$

$$\alpha = \frac{2d(a+c)+(2c(b+d)}{(a+c)(b+d)}$$

RIB, $a$ impenetrant

As CIB, $a$ impenetrant, substituting $b$ for $a$, $a$ for $b$, $d$ for $c$, and $c$ for $d$ in the formulae.

CBI, $a$ impenetrant

$$p = \frac{3c(b+d)-d(a+c)}{d(a+c)+3c(b+d)}$$

$$\alpha = \frac{d(a+c)+3c(b+d)}{2(a+c)(b+d)}$$

RBI, $a$ impenetrant

$$p = \frac{2d(a+c)}{d(a+c)+3c(b+d)}$$

$$\alpha = \frac{d(a+c)+3c(b+d)}{2(a+c)(b+d)}$$

CIB, $A'$ impenetrant

$$p = \frac{2b(a+c)-a(b+d)}{b(a+c)+a(b+d)}$$

$$\alpha = \frac{2b(a+c)+2a(b+d)}{3(a+c)(b+d)}$$

RIB, $A'$ impenetrant

As CIB, $A'$ impenetrant, substitute $b$ for $a$, $a$ for $b$, $d$ for $c$, and $c$ for $d$ in the formulae.

CBI, $A'$ impenetrant

As RBI, $a$ impenetrant, substitute $c$ for $a$, $d$ for $b$, $a$ for $c$, and $b$ for $d$ in the formulae.

RBI, $A'$ impenetrant

As CBI, $a$ impenetrant, substitute $c$ for $a$, $d$ for $b$, $a$ for $c$, and $b$ for $d$ in the formulae.

---

TABLE 6.5

Formulae for the terms of the matrices of the single backcross with one locus impenetrant

CIB, $a$ impenetrant

$$A = \frac{\alpha[2-\alpha+2\alpha p(1-p)]}{(1-p)p(2-\alpha p)[2-\alpha(1-p)]}$$

$$B = \frac{\alpha(2p-1)}{2(2-\alpha p)[2-\alpha(1-p)]}$$

$$D = \frac{1-\alpha p(1-p)}{\alpha(2-\alpha p)[2-\alpha(1-p)]}$$

CBI, $a$ impenetrant

$$A = \frac{\alpha[3-2\alpha+2\alpha p(1-p)]}{2(1+p)(1-p)[3-\alpha(1+p)][1-\alpha(1-p)]}$$

$$B = \frac{\alpha(2p-1)}{2[3-\alpha(1+p)][1-\alpha(1-p)]}$$

$$D = \frac{3-\alpha p(1-p)}{2\alpha[3-\alpha(1+p)][1-\alpha(1-p)]}$$

RBI, $a$ impenetrant

$$A = \frac{\alpha[3-2\alpha+2\alpha p(1-p)]}{2(2-p)p(1-\alpha p)[3-\alpha(1-p)]}$$

$$B = \frac{\alpha(2p-1)}{2(1-\alpha p)[3-\alpha(2-p)]}$$

$$D = \frac{3-2\alpha p(2-p)}{2\alpha(1-\alpha p)[3-\alpha(2-p)]}$$

CIB, $A'$ impenetrant

$$A = \frac{\alpha[6-5\alpha+2\alpha p(1-p)]}{2(2-p)(1+p)[2-\alpha(2-p)][2-\alpha(1+p)]}$$

$$B = \frac{\alpha(2p-1)}{2[2-\alpha(2-p)][2-\alpha(1+p)]}$$

$$D = \frac{3-2\alpha-\alpha p(1-p)}{[2-\alpha(2-p)][2-\alpha(1+p)]}$$

In the similar cases of repulsion phase with a recessive gene and of a dominant epistatic and impenetrant gene in both phases, the above formulae still hold, except that the class frequencies must be interchanged. Taking the last class as always the epistatic and defining $a+$ and $ab$ as equal to $++$ and $+b$ for the case of a dominant gene, the substitutions will be as follows:

| Epistatic and impenetrant gene | Phases | Frequencies | | |
|---|---|---|---|---|
| $a$ | Coupling | $a$ | $b$ | $c$ |
| $a$ | Repulsion | $b$ | $a$ | $c$ |
| $A'$ | Coupling | $b$ | $a$ | $c$ |
| $A'$ | Repulsion | $a$ | $b$ | $c$ |

All four cases will have the same variance. The matrix elements which lead to the calculation of this are shown in Table 6.6. The variance is then:

$$V = \frac{D}{n(AD - B^2)}.$$

The intercross will give rise to two situations, depending upon whether the affected gene is recessive or dominant. The initial estimate will be of $P$ as usual. The expectations for the intercross involving a recessive gene are:

| $++$ | $+b$ | $a+, ab$ |
|---|---|---|
| $\dfrac{3 - \alpha(1-P)}{4}$ | $\dfrac{1 - \alpha P}{4}$ | $\dfrac{\alpha}{4}$ |

Whence:

$$P = \frac{a+b-3b}{4c}, \qquad \alpha = \frac{4c}{n}.$$

The expectations for the intercross involving a dominant epistatic and impenetrant gene are:

| $++$ | $+b$ | $A'+, A'b$ |
|---|---|---|
| $\dfrac{3 - \alpha(2+P)}{4}$ | $\dfrac{1 - \alpha(1-P)}{4}$ | $\dfrac{3\alpha}{4}$ |

Whence:

$$P = \frac{9b+c-3a}{4c}, \qquad \alpha = \frac{4c}{3n}.$$

## TABLE 6.6

Formulae for the terms of the matrix of the testcross with gene $a$ epistatic and impenetrant

$$A = \frac{\alpha^2(2-\alpha)}{2(1-\alpha p)[1-\alpha(1-p)]}$$

$$B = \frac{\alpha(2p-1)}{2(1-\alpha p)[1-\alpha(1-p)]}$$

$$C = \frac{1-2\alpha p(1-p)}{2(1-\alpha p)[1-\alpha(1-p)]}$$

The two situations will have different matrices and these are shown in Tables 6.7 and 6.8. The variance is then:

$$V = \frac{D}{4nP(AD-B^2)}.$$

## TABLE 6.7

Formulae for the terms of the matrix of the intercross with a recessive epistatic and impenetrant gene

$$A = \frac{\alpha^2(4-\alpha)}{4(1-\alpha P)[3-\alpha(1-P)]}$$

$$B = \frac{\alpha(4P-1)}{4(1-\alpha P)[3-\alpha(1-P)]}$$

$$D = \frac{3-4\alpha P(1-P)}{4\alpha(1-\alpha P)[3-\alpha(1-P)]}$$

## TABLE 6.8

Formulae for the terms of the matrix of the intercross with a dominant epistatic and impenetrant gene

$$A = \frac{\alpha^2(4-3\alpha)}{4[3-\alpha(2+P)][1-\alpha(1-P)]}$$

$$B = \frac{\alpha(4P-1)}{4[3-\alpha(2+P)][1-\alpha(1-P)]}$$

$$D = \frac{9-8\alpha+4\alpha P(1+P)}{4\alpha[3-\alpha(2+P)][1-\alpha(1-P)]}$$

The single backcross presents the usual diversity of situations. There are eight possibilities but four of these are duplicates of the other four for computational purposes. These can be dealt with by appropriate substitution of frequencies. Table 6.9 gives the relevant estimating formulae for the four distinguishable situations and indicates the substitutions to be made for the others.

The various crosses will have matrix elements as shown in Table 6.10. Only the four distinguishable situations are

TABLE 6.9

Estimation of the crossover fraction and penetrance for the single backcross with a single epistatic and impenetrant locus

---

CIB, $a$ impenetrant

$$p = \frac{b+c-a}{2c}, \qquad \alpha = \frac{4c}{n}$$

RIB, $a$ impenetrant
As CIB, $a$ impenetrant, substitute $b$ for $a$, $a$ for $b$, and $c$ for $c$ in the formulae.

CBI, $a$ impenetrant

$$p = \frac{3b+c-a}{2c}, \qquad \alpha = \frac{2c}{n}$$

RBI, $a$ impenetrant

$$p = \frac{a+c-3b}{2c}, \qquad \alpha = \frac{2c}{n}$$

CIB, $A'$ impenetrant

$$p = \frac{a+c-b}{c}, \qquad \alpha = \frac{4c}{3n}$$

RIB, $A'$ impenetrant
As CIB, $A'$ impenetrant, substitute $b$ for $a$, $a$ for $b$, and $c$ for $c$ in the formulae.
CBI, $A'$ impenetrant
As RBI, $a$ impenetrant, substitute $a$ for $a$, $b$ for $b$, and $c$ for $c$ in the formulae.
RBI, $A'$ impenetrant
As CBI, $a$ impenetrant, substitute $a$ for $a$, $b$ for $b$, and $c$ for $c$ in the formulae.

---

TABLE 6.10

Formulae for the terms of the matrices of the single backcross with a single epistatic and impenetrant gene

---

CIB, $a$ impenetrant

$$A = \frac{\alpha^2(4-\alpha)}{4(2-\alpha p)[2-\alpha(1-p)]}$$

$$B = \frac{\alpha(2p-1)}{2(2-\alpha p)[2-\alpha(1-p)]}$$

$$D = \frac{1-\alpha p(1-p)}{\alpha(2-\alpha p)[2-\alpha(1-p)]}$$

CBI, $a$ impenetrant

$$A = \frac{\alpha^2(2-\alpha)}{4[3-\alpha(1+p)][1-\alpha(1-p)]}$$

$$B = \frac{\alpha(2p-1)}{2[3-\alpha(1+p)][1-\alpha(1+p)]}$$

$$D = \frac{3-2\alpha p(1-p)}{2[3-\alpha(1+p)][1-\alpha(1-p)]}$$

RBI, $a$ impenetrant

$$A = \frac{\alpha^2(4-3\alpha)}{4(1-\alpha p)[3-\alpha(2-p)]}$$

$$B = \frac{\alpha(2p-1)}{2(1-\alpha p)[3-\alpha(2-p)]}$$

$$D = \frac{3-2\alpha p(1-p)}{4\alpha(1-\alpha p)[3-\alpha(2-p)]}$$

CIB, $A'$ impenetrant

$$A = \frac{\alpha^2(4-3\alpha)}{4[2-\alpha(2-p)][2-\alpha(1+p)]}$$

$$B = \frac{\alpha(2p-1)}{2[2-\alpha(2-p)][2-\alpha(1+p)]}$$

$$D = \frac{3-2\alpha-\alpha p(1-p)}{\alpha[2-\alpha(2-p)][2-\alpha(1+p)]}$$

---

presented since the other four will have the same elements as the cross which they duplicate. The variance is then:

$$V = \frac{D}{n(AD-B^2)}.$$

When the impenetrance and the epistasis are due to different genes, independent estimation of $p$ and $\alpha$ is impossible if segregations of only one phase are available. However, when segregations of opposite phase are available, estimates can be made, subject to a qualification. This is that the value of $p$ and $\alpha$ are assumed to be identical for both segregations. This is usually taken to be true for $p$ but, of course, cannot be taken for granted for $\alpha$. The penetrance does vary between samples but the magnitude can possibly be minimized by experimenting with reciprocal crosses from the same generation, stock or strain. On the assumption that the penetrance in the two segregations are sensibly comparable, the expectations for coupling and repulsion backcrosses for gene $a$ impenetrant and gene $b$ epistatic are:

|  | Coupling | | Repulsion | |
|---|---|---|---|---|
|  | ++ | $a+$ | ++ | $a+$ |
| Expectation | $\dfrac{1-\alpha p}{2}$ | $\dfrac{\alpha p}{2}$ | $\dfrac{1-\alpha(1-p)}{2}$ | $\dfrac{\alpha(1-p)}{2}$ |
| Observations | $a$ | $b$ | $c$ | $d$ |

The epistatic classes ($+b$ and $ab$) contribute no information and these are ignored. To keep the analysis as simple as possible, equal numbers should be examined in the two segregations. The set of expectations can be seen to be identical to the coupling testcross in the absence of epistasis. For purposes of estimation, it is merely necessary to interchange the frequencies of the two middle classes ($c$ for $b$ and $b$ for $c$), whence the formulae for $p$ and $\alpha$ given earlier can be used. This set of expectations has two df. The total $n$ will be for summation over all four classes. The variances will be the same as for the testcross in the absence of epistatis.

Four situations can occur, depending whether the recessive or dominant gene is impenetrant or epistatic. Basically, these are identical, except that the various phenotypic classes will have different, yet interchangeable, frequencies. When $B'$ is epistatic, the two distinguishable classes will be $+b^+$ and $ab^+$ and these will be taken as equivalent to $++$ and $a+$. Always considering the coupling segregation first, the observed frequencies as designated above should be interchanged for the frequencies $a$, $b$, $c$, and $d$ of the coupling testcross as follows:

| Impenetrant | Epistatic | Class frequencies | | | |
|:---:|:---:|:---:|:---:|:---:|:---:|
| $a$ | $b$ | $a$ | $c$ | $b$ | $d$ |
| $a$ | $B'$ | $c$ | $a$ | $d$ | $b$ |
| $A'$ | $b$ | $d$ | $b$ | $c$ | $a$ |
| $A'$ | $B'$ | $b$ | $d$ | $a$ | $c$ |

The above form of analysis can be extended to the intercross and single backcross. Fairly simple estimating formulae can be derived for $p$ but not for the mean $\alpha$. The expressions for the information are complicated and, in view of the fact that these situations are only of marginal importance, will not be given. It seems worth while to note that many problems of this nature can be tackled by combination of segregations of opposite linkage phase, despite the fact that the statistical efficiency is probably low.

## Two Impenetrant Loci

The analysis of segregations in which both genes are impenetrant proceeds similarly to that of the foregoing section, except for the introduction of an extra parameter. The impenetrance of locus $b$ will be denoted by $\beta$. The expectations for the coupling testcross with two recessive impenetrant genes are:

| | $++$ | $+b$ | $a+$ | $ab$ |
|---|:---:|:---:|:---:|:---:|
| Exp. | $\dfrac{2-\alpha-\beta+\alpha\beta(1-p)}{2}$ | $\dfrac{\beta-\alpha\beta(1-p)}{2}$ | $\dfrac{\alpha-\alpha\beta(1-p)}{2}$ | $\dfrac{\alpha\beta(1-p)}{2}$ |
| Obser. | $a$ | $b$ | $c$ | $d$ |

$$1-p = \frac{dn}{2(b+d)(c+d)}, \qquad \alpha = \frac{2(c+d)}{n}, \qquad \beta = \frac{2(b+d)}{n}.$$

The testcross generates six different situations depending upon phase and whether the impenetrant genes are recessive or dominant. The same estimating formulae can be used in conjunction with the appropriate interchange of phenotype classes. It should be particularly noted, however, that analysis of segregations 1, 4, and 5 gives an estimate of $1-p$ while segregations 2, 3, and 6 give direct estimates of $p$. Keeping this in mind, the following substitutions should be made:

| | Impenetrance genes | | Phase | Frequencies | | | |
|---|---|---|---|---|---|---|---|
| 1. | $a$ | $b$ | Coupling | $a$ | $b$ | $c$ | $d$ |
| 2. | $a$ | $b$ | Repulsion | $a$ | $b$ | $c$ | $d$ |
| 3. | $A'$ | $b$ | Coupling | $c$ | $d$ | $a$ | $b$ |
| 4. | $A'$ | $b$ | Repulsion | $c$ | $d$ | $a$ | $b$ |
| 5. | $A'$ | $B'$ | Coupling | $d$ | $c$ | $b$ | $a$ |
| 6. | $A'$ | $B'$ | Repulsion | $d$ | $c$ | $b$ | $a$ |

TABLE 6.11

Formulae for the terms of the matrix of the testcross with two impenetrant genes

$$A = \frac{\alpha\beta}{2}\left(\frac{\alpha\beta(1-C)+\alpha A}{A(1-C)} + \frac{1}{(1-B)(1-p)}\right)$$

$$B = \frac{\alpha\beta(2p-1)}{2A(1-C)}$$

$$C = \frac{\alpha\beta(2p-1)}{2A(1-C)}$$

$$D = \frac{2-\beta-2C(1-B)}{2\alpha A(1-C)}$$

$$E = \frac{2p-1}{2A}$$

$$D = \frac{2-\alpha-2B(1-C)}{2\alpha A(1-B)}$$

Where $A = 2-\alpha-\beta+\alpha\beta(1-p)$,     $B = \beta(1-p)$    and    $C = \alpha(1-p)$.

The matrix elements for the calculation of the variance are given by Table 6.11. The variance is then:

$$V = \frac{DF - E^2}{n[A(DF - E^2) + B(2CE - BF) - C^2 D]}.$$

Bailey (1950) has derived the following formulae for the variance, based on the amount of realized information:

$$V = \frac{dn[n(d^2 + bc) - d(b+d)(d+c)]}{4(b+d)^3 (d+c)^3},$$

substitution of frequencies being made according to the type of cross.

The intercross generates three different situations, according to the particular combination of recessiveness and dominance of the impenetrant genes. When both impenetrant genes are recessive, the expectations are:

| ++ | +b | a+ | ab |
|----|----|----|----|
| $\dfrac{4 - \alpha - \beta + \alpha\beta P}{4}$ | $\dfrac{\beta(1 - \alpha P)}{4}$ | $\dfrac{\alpha(1 - \beta P)}{4}$ | $\dfrac{\alpha\beta P}{4}$ |

Whence:

$$P = \frac{dn}{4(b+d)(c+d)}, \qquad \alpha = \frac{4(c+d)}{n}, \qquad \beta = \frac{4(b+d)}{n}.$$

When one gene $(A')$ is dominant and the other recessive $(b)$, the expectations are:

| $A'+$ | $A'b$ | ++ | +b |
|-------|-------|----|----|
| $\dfrac{\alpha[3 - \beta(1-P)]}{4}$ | $\dfrac{\alpha\beta(1-P)}{4}$ | $\dfrac{4 - 3\alpha - \beta[1 - \alpha(1-P)]}{4}$ | $\dfrac{\beta[1 - \alpha(1-P)]}{4}$ |

Whence:

$$P = 1 - \frac{3bn}{4(a+b)(b+d)}, \qquad \alpha = \frac{4(a+b)}{3n}, \qquad \beta = \frac{4(b+d)}{n}.$$

When both of the impenetrant genes are dominant, the expectations are:

| $A'B'$ | $A'b$ | $++$ | $+b$ |

$$\frac{\alpha\beta(2+P)}{4} \quad \frac{\alpha[3-\beta(2+P)]}{4} \quad \frac{\beta[3-\alpha(2+P)]}{4} \quad \frac{4-3\alpha-3\beta+\alpha\beta(2+P)}{4}$$

Whence:

$$P = 2 - \frac{3an}{4(a+b)(a+c)}, \qquad \alpha = \frac{4(a+b)}{3n}, \qquad \beta = \frac{4(a+c)}{3n}.$$

The matrix elements for the calculation of the variances of these three situations are shown by Tables 6.12, 6.13, and 6.14. The variance is then:

$$V = \frac{DF-E^2}{4nP[A(DF-E^2)+B(2CE-BF)-C^2D]}.$$

The single backcross presents a variety of situations but the numbers of different cases can be reduced by stipulating that the impenetrant gene assorting in the 3 : 1 ratio is invariably represented by locus $a$. There are then eight cases to consider,

TABLE 6.12

Formulae for the terms of the matrix of the intercross with two recessive impenetrant genes

$$A = \frac{\alpha\beta}{4}\left(\frac{\alpha\beta(1-\alpha P)+\alpha A}{A(1-\alpha P)} + \frac{1}{(1-\beta P)P}\right)$$

$$B = \frac{\alpha\beta(4P-1)}{4A(1-\alpha P)}$$

$$C = \frac{\alpha\beta(4P-1)}{4A(1-\beta P)}$$

$$D = \frac{4-\beta-4\alpha P(1-\beta P)}{4\alpha A(1-\alpha P)}$$

$$E = \frac{4P-1}{4A}$$

$$F = \frac{4-\alpha-4\beta P(1-\alpha P)}{4\beta A(1-\beta P)}$$

Where $A = 4-\alpha-\beta+\alpha\beta P$.

## TABLE 6.13

Formulae for the terms of the matrix of the intercross with one dominant $(A')$ and one recessive $(b)$ impenetrant gene

$$A = \frac{\alpha\beta}{4}\left(\frac{\alpha\beta(1-C)+\alpha A}{A(1-C)} + \frac{3}{(3-B)(1-P)}\right)$$

$$B = \frac{\alpha\beta(4P-1)}{4A(1-C)}$$

$$C = \frac{\alpha\beta(4P-1)}{4A(1-B)}$$

$$D = \frac{12-3\beta-12\alpha(1-P)+4\alpha\beta(1-P)^2}{4\alpha A(1-C)}$$

$$E = \frac{4P-1}{4A}$$

$$F = \frac{12-9\alpha-4\beta(1-P)+4\alpha\beta(1-P)}{4\alpha\beta(3-B)}$$

Where: $A = 4-3\alpha-\beta[1-\alpha(1-P)]$, $B = \beta(1-P)$ and $C = \alpha(1-P)$.

## TABLE 6.14

Formulae for the terms of the matrix of the intercross for two dominant impenetrant genes

$$A = \frac{\alpha\beta}{4}\left(\frac{\alpha\beta(3-C)+\alpha A}{A(3-C)} + \frac{3}{(2+P)(3-B)}\right)$$

$$B = \frac{\alpha\beta(4P-1)}{4A(3-C)}$$

$$C = \frac{\alpha\beta(4P-1)}{4A(3-B)}$$

$$D = \frac{36-27\beta-12\alpha(2+P)+4\alpha\beta(2+P)}{4\alpha A(3-C)}$$

$$E = \frac{4P-1}{4A}$$

$$F = \frac{36-27\alpha-12\beta(2+P)+4\alpha\beta(2+P)^2}{4\beta A(3-B)}$$

Where: $A = 4-3\alpha-3\beta+\alpha\beta(2+P)$, $B = \beta(2+P)$ and $C = \alpha(2+P)$.

taking into account phase and dominance. The expectations for the coupling phase with two recessive impenetrant genes are:

$$++ \qquad\qquad +b \qquad\qquad a+ \qquad\qquad ab$$

$$\frac{4-\alpha-2\beta+\alpha\beta(1-p)}{4} \quad \frac{\beta[2-\alpha(1-p)]}{4} \quad \frac{\alpha[1-\beta(1-p)]}{4} \quad \frac{\alpha\beta(1-p)}{4}$$

Whence:

$$1-p=\frac{dn}{2(b+d)(c+d)}, \qquad \alpha=\frac{4(c+d)}{n}, \qquad \beta=\frac{2(b+d)}{n}.$$

The repulsion phase with two recessive impenetrant genes has similar expectations to the above and the same formulae may be used, except that the estimate is now of $p$, instead of $1-p$.

The expectations for the coupling phase with two dominant impenetrant genes are:

$$A'B' \qquad\qquad A'+ \qquad\qquad +B' \qquad\qquad ++$$

$$\frac{\alpha\beta(2-p)}{4} \quad \frac{\alpha[3-\beta(2-p)]}{4} \quad \frac{\beta[2-\alpha(2-p)]}{4} \quad \frac{4-3\alpha-2\beta+\alpha\beta(2-p)}{4}$$

Whence:

$$2-p=\frac{3an}{2(a+b)(a+c)}, \qquad \alpha=\frac{4(a+b)}{3n}, \qquad \beta=\frac{2(a+c)}{n}.$$

The corresponding repulsion phase has similar expectations and the same formulae can be used, except that the estimate will be of $1+p$, instead of $2-p$.

The coupling phase with one recessive gene $(b)$ and one dominant gene $(A')$ has the expectations:

$$A'+ \qquad\qquad A'b \qquad\qquad ++ \qquad\qquad +b$$

$$\frac{\alpha[3-\beta(1+p)]}{4} \quad \frac{\alpha\beta(1+p)}{4} \quad \frac{4-3\alpha-2\beta+\alpha\beta(1+p)}{4} \quad \frac{\beta[2-\alpha(1+p)]}{4}$$

Whence:

$$1+p=\frac{3bn}{2(a+b)(b+d)}, \qquad \alpha=\frac{4(a+b)}{3n}, \qquad \beta=\frac{2(b+d)}{n}.$$

The corresponding repulsion phase has similar expectations and the same formulae may be used, except the estimate will be of $2-p$, instead of $1+p$.

The obverse case of coupling where the recessive gene is $a$ and the dominant gene is $B'$ has the expectations:

| $+B'$ | $++$ | $aB'$ | $a+$ |
|---|---|---|---|
| $\dfrac{\alpha(2-\beta p)}{4}$ | $\dfrac{\alpha\beta p}{4}$ | $\dfrac{4-2\alpha-\beta+\alpha\beta p}{4}$ | $\dfrac{\beta(1-\alpha p)}{4}$ |

Whence:

$$p = \frac{bn}{2(a+b)(b+d)}, \qquad \alpha - \frac{2(a+b)}{n}, \qquad \beta = \frac{4(b+d)}{n}.$$

The repulsion phase has similar expectations and the above formulae may be used, except the estimation will be of $1-p$, instead of $p$.

TABLE 6.15

Formulae for the terms of the matrix of the single backcross for the two recessive impenetrant genes

$$A = \frac{\alpha\beta}{4}\left(\frac{\alpha\beta(2-C)+\alpha A}{A(2-C)} + \frac{1}{(1-p)(1-B)}\right)$$

$$B = \frac{\alpha\beta(2p-1)}{2A(2-C)}$$

$$C = \frac{\alpha\beta(2p-1)}{2A(1-B)}$$

$$D = \frac{2-\beta-\alpha(1-p)+\alpha\beta(1-p)^2}{\alpha A(2-p)}$$

$$E = \frac{2p-1}{2A}$$

$$F = \frac{4-\alpha-4\beta(1-p)+2\alpha\beta(1-p)^2}{2\beta A(1-B)}$$

Where: $A = 4-\alpha-2\beta+\alpha\beta(1-p)$, $\quad B = \beta(1-p)$ and $C = \alpha(1-p)$.
For repulsion phase, substitute $p$ for $1-p$.

## TABLE 6.16

Formulae for the terms of the matrix of the single backcross for two dominant impenetrant genes

$$A = \frac{\alpha\beta}{4}\left(\frac{\alpha\beta(2-C)+\beta A}{A(2-C)} + \frac{3}{(2-p)(3-B)}\right)$$

$$B = \frac{\alpha\beta(2p-1)}{2A(2-C)}$$

$$C = \frac{\alpha\beta(2p-1)}{2A(3-B)}$$

$$D = \frac{6-3\beta-3\alpha(2-p)+\alpha\beta(2-p)}{\alpha A(2-C)}$$

$$E = \frac{2p-1}{2A}$$

$$F = \frac{12-9\alpha-4\beta(2-p)+2\alpha\beta(2-p)^2}{2\beta A(3-B)}$$

Where: $A = 4-3\alpha-2\beta+\alpha\beta(2-p)$, $\quad B = \beta(2-p)$ $\quad$ and $\quad C = \alpha(2-p)$.

For repulsion phase, substitute $1+p$ for $2-p$.

## TABLE 6.17

Formulae for the terms of the matrix of the single backcross with one recessive gene $(b)$ and one dominant gene $(A')$ impenetrant

$$A = \frac{\alpha\beta}{4}\left(\frac{\alpha\beta(2-C)+\beta A}{A(2-C)} + \frac{3}{(1+p)(3-B)}\right)$$

$$B = \frac{\alpha\beta(2p-1)}{2A(2-C)}$$

$$C = \frac{\alpha\beta(2p-1)}{2A(3-B)}$$

$$D = \frac{6-3\beta-3\alpha(1+p)+\alpha\beta(1+p)}{\alpha A(2-C)}$$

$$E = \frac{2p-1}{2A}$$

$$F = \frac{12-9\alpha-4\beta(1+p)+2\alpha\beta(2-p)^2}{\beta A(3-B)}$$

Where: $A = 4-3\alpha-2\beta+\alpha\beta(1+p)$, $\quad B = \beta(1+p)$ $\quad$ and $\quad C = \alpha(1+p)$.

For repulsion phase, substitute $2-p$ for $1+p$.

TABLE 6.18

Formulae for the terms of the matrix of the single backcross with one recessive gene (a) and one dominant gene ($B'$) impenetrant

$$A = \frac{\alpha\beta}{4}\left(\frac{\alpha\beta(2-B)+\beta A}{A(2-B)} + \frac{1}{p(1-C)}\right)$$

$$B = \frac{\alpha\beta(2p-1)}{2A(2-B)}$$

$$C = \frac{\alpha\beta(2p-1)}{2A(1-C)}$$

$$D = \frac{4-\beta-2\alpha p(2-\beta p)}{2\alpha A(1-C)}$$

$$E = \frac{2p-1}{2A}$$

$$F = \frac{2-\alpha-\beta p(1-\alpha p)}{\beta A(2-B)}$$

Where: $A = 4-2\alpha-\beta+\alpha\beta p$,    $B = \beta p$   and   $C = \alpha p$.

For repulsion phase, substitute $1-p$ for $p$.

The matrix elements for the various crosses are shown by Tables 6.15, 6.16., 6.17, and 6.18. Note the substitutions which are necessary to transform the coupling matrix into that for repulsion. The variance is then:

$$V = \frac{DF-E^2}{n[A(DF-E^2)+B(2CE-BF)-C^2D]}.$$

# CHAPTER 7

# Estimation with Inviability and Impenetrance

The analysis of segregations in which an allele at one locus displays inviability while the allele at the other displays impenetrance presents much the same problems as for impenetrance alone. The expectations may seem more complicated but the estimating formulae are either identical or analogous to many of those given earlier. Locus $a$ will be assumed to be impenetrant and locus $b$ the inviable. The expectations for the coupling testcross with two recessive genes are:

| | $++$ | $+b$ | $a+$ | $ab$ |
|---|---|---|---|---|
| | $\dfrac{1-\alpha p}{1+u}$ | $\dfrac{u[1-\alpha(1-p)]}{1+u}$ | $\dfrac{\alpha p}{1+u}$ | $\dfrac{\alpha u(1-p)}{1+u}$ |
| Observations | $a$ | $b$ | $c$ | $d$ |

Whence:

$$p = \frac{c(b+d)}{d(a+c)+c(b+d)}, \qquad \alpha = \frac{d(a+c)+c(b+d)}{(a+c)(b+d)}, \qquad u = \frac{b+d}{a+c}.$$

The testcross involves eight cases, depending upon phase and whether a recessive or dominant gene is impenetrant or semi-viable. The expectations are identical in each case but occur for different phenotype classes. This means that the same estimating formulae can be used but with interchanges of observations. It should be noted that segregations 1, 4, 6, and 7 lead directly to an estimate of $p$ while 2, 3, 5, and 8 produce an estimate of $1-p$. Bearing this in mind, the following substitutions should be made:

| | Impenetrant | Semi-viable | Phase | Frequencies | | | |
|---|---|---|---|---|---|---|---|
| 1 | $a$ | $b$ | Coupling | $a$ | $b$ | $c$ | $d$ |
| 2 | $a$ | $b$ | Repulsion | $a$ | $b$ | $c$ | $d$ |
| 3 | $a$ | $B'$ | Coupling | $b$ | $a$ | $d$ | $c$ |
| 4 | $a$ | $B'$ | Repulsion | $b$ | $a$ | $d$ | $c$ |
| 5 | $A'$ | $b$ | Coupling | $c$ | $d$ | $a$ | $b$ |
| 6 | $A'$ | $b$ | Repulsion | $c$ | $d$ | $a$ | $b$ |
| 7 | $A'$ | $B'$ | Coupling | $d$ | $c$ | $b$ | $a$ |
| 8 | $A'$ | $B'$ | Repulsion | $d$ | $c$ | $b$ | $a$ |

All of these cases have the same variance and the matrix elements are presented in Table 7.1. The variance is then:

$$V = \frac{D}{n(AD - B^2)}.$$

The intercross gives rise to four situations, according to the particular combination of recessive and dominance of the

TABLE 7.1

Formulae for the terms of the matrix of the testcross with one gene impenetrant and one gene inviable

$$A = \frac{\alpha}{1+u}\left(\frac{1}{p(1-\alpha p)} + \frac{u}{(1-p)[1-\alpha(1-p)]}\right)$$

$$B = \frac{1}{1+u}\left(\frac{1}{1-\alpha p} - \frac{u}{1-\alpha(1-p)}\right)$$

$$C = 0$$

$$D = \frac{1}{\alpha(1-p)}\left(\frac{p}{1-\alpha p} + \frac{u(1-p)}{1-\alpha(1-p)}\right)$$

$$E = 0$$

$$F = \frac{1}{u(1+u)^2}$$

impenetrant or inviable genes. For the case of two recessive genes, the expectations are:

| ++ | +b | a+ | ab |
|---|---|---|---|
| $\dfrac{3-\alpha(1-P)}{3+u}$ | $\dfrac{u(1-\alpha P)}{3+u}$ | $\dfrac{\alpha(1-P)}{3+u}$ | $\dfrac{\alpha u P}{3+u}$ |

Whence:

$$P = \frac{d(a+c)}{d(a+c)+3c(b+d)}, \quad \alpha = \frac{d(a+c)+3c(b+d)}{(a+c)(b+d)}, \quad u = \frac{3(b+d)}{a+c}.$$

For the case of gene $a$ impenetrant and $B'$ inviable, the expectations are:

| +B' | +B' | a+ | a+ |
|---|---|---|---|
| $\dfrac{u[3-\alpha(1-P)]}{1+3u}$ | $\dfrac{1-\alpha P}{1+3u}$ | $\dfrac{\alpha u(1-P)}{1+3u}$ | $\dfrac{\alpha P}{1+3u}$ |

Whence:

$$P = \frac{d(a+c)}{d(a+c)+3c(b+d)}, \quad \alpha = \frac{d(a+c)+3c(b+d)}{(a+c)(b+d)}, \quad u = \frac{a+c}{3(b+d)}.$$

For the case of gene $A'$ impenetrant and $b$ inviable, the expectations are:

| +A' | A'b | ++ | +b |
|---|---|---|---|
| $\dfrac{\alpha(2+P)}{3+u}$ | $\dfrac{\alpha u(1-P)}{3+u}$ | $\dfrac{3-\alpha(2+P)}{3+u}$ | $\dfrac{u[1-\alpha(1-P)]}{3+u}$ |

Whence:

$$P = \frac{a(b+3d)-2bc}{b(a+c)+3a(b+d)}, \quad \alpha = \frac{b(a+c)-3a(b+d)}{3(a+c)(b+d)}, \quad u = \frac{3(b+d)}{a+c}.$$

For the case of gene $A'$ impenetrant and $B'$ inviable, the expectations are:

| A'B' | A'+ | +B' | ++ |
|---|---|---|---|
| $\dfrac{\alpha u(2+P)}{1+3u}$ | $\dfrac{\alpha(1-P)}{1+3u}$ | $\dfrac{u[3-\alpha(2+P)]}{1+3u}$ | $\dfrac{1-\alpha(1-P)}{1+3u}$ |

Whence:

$$P = \frac{a(b+3d)-2bc}{b(a+c)+3a(b+d)}, \qquad \alpha = \frac{b(a+c)-3a(b+d)}{3(a+c)(b+d)}, \qquad u = \frac{a+c}{3(b+d)}.$$

TABLE 7.2

Formulae for the terms of the matrix of the intercross with a recessive impenetrant gene and a recessive inviable gene

$$A = \frac{\alpha}{3+u}\left(\frac{3}{(1-P)[3-\alpha(1-P)]} + \frac{u}{P(1-\alpha P)}\right)$$

$$B = \frac{1}{3+u}\left(\frac{u}{1-\alpha P} - \frac{3}{3-\alpha(1-P)}\right)$$

$$C = 0$$

$$D = \frac{1}{\alpha(3+u)}\left(\frac{uP}{1-\alpha P} + \frac{3(1-P)}{3-\alpha(1-P)}\right)$$

$$E = 0$$

$$F = \frac{1}{u(3+u)^2}$$

TABLE 7.3

Formulae for the terms of the matrix of the intercross with a recessive impenetrant gene ($a$) and a dominant inviable ($B'$)

$$A = \frac{\alpha}{1+3u}\left(\frac{3u}{(1-P)[3-\alpha(1-P)]} + \frac{1}{P(1-\alpha P)}\right)$$

$$B = \frac{1}{1+3u}\left(\frac{1}{1-\alpha P} - \frac{3u}{3-\alpha(1-P)}\right)$$

$$C = 0$$

$$D = \frac{1}{\alpha(1+3u)}\left(\frac{P}{1-\alpha P} + \frac{3u(1-P)}{3-\alpha(1-P)}\right)$$

$$E = 0$$

$$F = \frac{1}{u(1+3u)^2}$$

TABLE 7.4

Formulae for the terms of the matrix of the intercross with a dominant impenetrant gene ($A'$) and a recessive inviable gene ($b$)

$$A = \frac{\alpha}{3+u}\left(\frac{3}{(2+P)[3-\alpha(2+P)]} + \frac{u}{(1-P)[1-\alpha(1-P)]}\right)$$

$$B = \frac{1}{3+u}\left(\frac{3}{3-\alpha(2+P)} - \frac{u}{1-\alpha(1-P)}\right)$$

$$C = 0$$

$$D = \frac{1}{\alpha(3+u)}\left(\frac{3(2+P)}{3-\alpha(2+P)} + \frac{u(1-P)}{1-\alpha(1-P)}\right)$$

$$E = 0$$

$$F = \frac{1}{u(3+u)^2}$$

TABLE 7.5

Formulae for the terms of the matrix of the intercross with a dominant impenetrant gene and a dominant inviable gene

$$A = \frac{\alpha}{1+3u}\left(\frac{3u}{(2+P)[3-\alpha(2+P)]} + \frac{1}{(1-P)[1-\alpha(1-P)]}\right)$$

$$B = \frac{1}{1+3u}\left(\frac{3u}{3-\alpha(2+P)} - \frac{1}{1-\alpha(1-P)}\right)$$

$$C = 0$$

$$D = \frac{1}{\alpha(1+3u)}\left(\frac{1-P}{1-\alpha(1-P)} + \frac{3u(2+P)}{3-\alpha(2+P)}\right)$$

$$E = 0$$

$$F = \frac{3}{u(1+3u)^2}$$

In each instance, the estimate will be of $P$ and $p$ must be derived by the usual relations. The variance for each case will differ slightly as shown by the terms of the respective matrices given in Tables 7.2, 7.3, 7.4, and 7.5. The variance is then:

$$V = \frac{D}{4nP(AD - B^2)}.$$

TABLE 7.6

Estimation of the crossover fraction, penetrance and viability for the single backcross

---

CIB, $a$ impenetrant, $b$ inviable

$$p = \frac{c(b+d)}{d(a+c)+c(b+d)}, \qquad \alpha = \frac{2d(a+c)+2c(b+d)}{(a+c)(b+d)}, \qquad u = \frac{b+d}{a+c}$$

RIB, $a$ impenetrant, $b$ inviable

$$p = \frac{d(a+c)}{d(a+c)+c(b+d)}$$

$\alpha$ and $u$ same as above

CBI, $a$ impenetrant, $b$ inviable

$$p = \frac{3c(b+d)-d(a+c)}{d(a+c)+3c(b+d)}, \qquad \alpha = \frac{d(a+c)+3c(b+d)}{2(a+c)(b+d)}, \qquad u = \frac{3(b+d)}{a+c}$$

RBI, $a$ impenetrant, $b$ inviable

$$p = \frac{2d(a+c)}{d(a+c)+3c(b+d)}$$

$\alpha$ and $u$ same as above

CIB, $a$ impenetrant, $B'$ inviable
  $p$ and $\alpha$ same as CIB, $a$ impenetrant, $b$ inviable, and:

$$u = \frac{a+c}{b+d}$$

RIB, $a$ impenetrant, $B'$ inviable
  $p$ and $\alpha$ same as RIB, $a$ impenetrant, $b$ inviable and $u$ same as above

CBI, $a$ impenetrant, $B'$ inviable
  $p$ and $\alpha$ same as CBI, $a$ impenetrant, $b$ inviable, and:

$$u = \frac{a+c}{3(b+d)}$$

Table 7.6—*(Continued)*

RBI, $a$ impenetrant, $B'$ inviable
  $p$ and $\alpha$ same as RBI, $a$ impenetrant, $b$ inviable and $u$ same as above

CIB, $A'$ impenetrant, $b$ inviable

$$p = \frac{2b(a+c) - a(b+d)}{b(a+c) + a(b+d)}, \qquad \alpha = \frac{2b(a+c) + 2a(b+d)}{3(a+c)(b+d)}, \qquad u = \frac{b+d}{a+c}$$

RIB, $A'$ impenetrant, $b$ inviable

$$p = \frac{2a(b+d) - b(a+c)}{b(a+c) + a(b+d)}$$

$\alpha$ and $u$ same as above

CBI, $A'$ impenetrant, $b$ inviable

$$p = \frac{2b(a+c)}{b(a+c) + 3a(b+d)}, \qquad \alpha = \frac{b(a+c) + 3a(b+d)}{2(a+c)(b+d)}, \qquad u = \frac{3(b+d)}{a+c}$$

RBI, $A'$ impenetrant, $b$ inviable

$$p = \frac{3a(b+d) - b(a+c)}{b(a+c) + 3a(b+d)}$$

$\alpha$ and $u$ same as above

CBI, $A'$ impenetrant, $B'$ inviable
  $p$ and $\alpha$ same as CIB, $A'$ impenetrant, $b$ inviable, and:

$$u = \frac{a+c}{b+d}$$

RIB, $A'$ impenetrant, $B'$ inviable

$$p = \frac{2a(b+d) - b(a+c)}{b(a+c) + a(b+d)}$$

$\alpha$ and $u$ same as above

CBI, $A'$ impenetrant, $B'$ inviable
  $p$ and $\alpha$ same as CBI, $A'$ impenetrant, $b$ inviable, and:

$$u = \frac{a+c}{3(b+d)}$$

RBI, $A'$ impenetrant, $B'$ inviable

$$p = \frac{3a(b+d) - b(a+c)}{b(a+c) + 3a(b+d)}, \qquad \alpha = \frac{b(a+c) + 3a(b+d)}{2(a+c)(b+d)}, \qquad u = \frac{a+c}{3(b+d)}$$

## TABLE 7.7

Formulae for the terms of the matrix of the single backcross for various combinations of dominance, impenetrance, and viability

CIB, $a$ impenetrant, $b$ inviable

$$A = \frac{\alpha}{1+u}\left(\frac{1}{p(2-\alpha p)} + \frac{u}{(1-p)[2-\alpha(1-p)]}\right)$$

$$B = \frac{1}{1+u}\left(\frac{1}{2-\alpha p} - \frac{u}{2-\alpha(1-p)}\right)$$

$$C = 0$$

$$D = \frac{1}{\alpha(1+u)}\left(\frac{p}{2-\alpha p} + \frac{u(1-p)}{2-\alpha(1-p)}\right)$$

$$E = 0$$

$$F = \frac{1}{u(1+u)^2}$$

RIB, $a$ impenetrant, $b$ inviable

$$A = \frac{\alpha}{1+u}\left(\frac{1}{(1-p)[2-\alpha(1-p)]} + \frac{u}{p(2-\alpha p)}\right)$$

$$B = \frac{1}{1+u}\left(\frac{u}{2-\alpha p} - \frac{1}{2-\alpha(1-p)}\right)$$

$$C = 0$$

$$D = \frac{1}{\alpha(1+u)}\left(\frac{1-p}{2-\alpha(1-p)} + \frac{up}{2-\alpha p}\right)$$

$$E = 0$$

$$F = \frac{1}{u(1+u)^2}$$

CBI, $a$ impenetrant, $b$ inviable

$$A = \frac{\alpha}{3+u}\left(\frac{3}{(1+p)[3-\alpha(1+p)]} + \frac{u}{(1-p)[1-\alpha(1-p)]}\right)$$

$$B = \frac{1}{3+u}\left(\frac{3}{3-\alpha(1+p)} - \frac{u}{1-\alpha(1-p)}\right)$$

$$C = 0$$

Table 7.7—*(Continued)*

$$D = \frac{1}{\alpha(3+u)}\left(\frac{3(1+p)}{3-\alpha(1+p)} + \frac{u(1-p)}{1-\alpha(1-p)}\right)$$

$$E = 0$$

$$F = \frac{3}{u(3+u)^2}$$

RBI, *a* impenetrant, *b* inviable

$$A = \frac{\alpha}{3+u}\left(\frac{3}{(2-p)[3-\alpha(2-p)]} + \frac{u}{p(1-\alpha p)}\right)$$

$$B = \frac{1}{3+u}\left(\frac{u}{1-\alpha p} - \frac{3}{3-\alpha(2-p)}\right)$$

$$C = 0$$

$$D = \frac{1}{\alpha(3+u)}\left(\frac{3(2-p)}{3-\alpha(2-p)} + \frac{up}{1-\alpha p}\right)$$

$$E = 0$$

$$F = \frac{3}{u(3+u)^2}$$

CIB, *a* impenetrant, *B'* inviable
    Same as RIB, *a* impenetrant, *b* inviable

RIB, *a* impenetrant, *B'* inviable
    Same as CIB, *a* impenetrant, *b* inviable

CBI, *a* impenetrant, *B'* inviable

$$A = \frac{\alpha}{1+3u}\left(\frac{1}{(1-p)[1-\alpha(1-p)]} + \frac{3u}{(1+p)[3-\alpha(1+p)]}\right)$$

$$B = \frac{1}{1+3u}\left(\frac{3u}{3-\alpha(1+p)} - \frac{1}{1-\alpha(1-p)}\right)$$

$$C = 0$$

$$D = \frac{1}{\alpha(1+3u)}\left(\frac{1-p}{1-\alpha(1-p)} + \frac{3u(1+p)}{3-\alpha(1+p)}\right)$$

$$E = 0$$

$$F = \frac{3}{u(1+3u)^2}$$

Table 7.7—*(Continued)*

RBI, *a* impenetrant, $B'$ inviable

$$A = \frac{\alpha}{1+3u}\left(\frac{1}{p(1-\alpha p)} + \frac{3u}{(2-p)[3-\alpha(2-p)]}\right)$$

$$B = \frac{1}{1+3u}\left(\frac{1}{1-\alpha p} - \frac{3u}{3-\alpha(2-p)}\right)$$

$$C = 0$$

$$D = \frac{1}{\alpha(1+3u)}\left(\frac{p}{1-\alpha p} + \frac{3u(2-p)}{3-\alpha(2-p)}\right)$$

$$E = 0$$

$$F = \frac{3}{u(1+3u)^2}$$

CIB, $A'$ impenetrant, *b* inviable

$$A = \frac{\alpha}{1+u}\left(\frac{1}{(2-p)[2-\alpha(2-p)]} + \frac{u}{(1+p)[2-\alpha(1+p)]}\right)$$

$$B = \frac{1}{1+u}\left(\frac{u}{2-\alpha(1+p)} - \frac{1}{2-\alpha(2-p)}\right)$$

$$C = 0$$

$$D = \frac{1}{\alpha(1+u)}\left(\frac{2-p}{2-\alpha(2-p)} + \frac{u(1+p)}{2-\alpha(1+p)}\right)$$

$$E = 0$$

$$F = \frac{1}{u(1+u)^2}$$

RIB, $A'$ impenetrant, *b* inviable

$$A = \frac{\alpha}{1+u}\left(\frac{1}{(1+p)[2-\alpha(1+p)]} + \frac{u}{(2-p)[2-\alpha(2-p)]}\right)$$

$$B = \frac{1}{1+u}\left(\frac{1}{2-\alpha(1+p)} - \frac{u}{2-\alpha(2-p)}\right)$$

$$C = 0$$

$$D = \frac{1}{\alpha(1+u)}\left(\frac{1+p}{2-\alpha(1+p)} + \frac{u(2-p)}{2-\alpha(2-p)}\right)$$

$$E = 0$$

Table 7.7—(Continued)

$$F = \frac{1}{u(1+u)^2}$$

CBI, $A'$ impenetrant, $b$ inviable
  Same as RBI, $a$ impenetrant, $b$ inviable

RBI, $A'$ impenetrant, $b$ inviable
  Same as CBI, $a$ impenetrant, $b$ inviable

CIB, $A'$ impenetrant, $B'$ inviable
  Same as RIB, $A'$ impenetrant, $b$ inviable

RIB, $A'$ impenetrant, $B'$ inviable
  Same as CIB, $A'$ impenetrant, $b$ inviable

CBI, $A'$ impenetrant, $B'$ inviable
  Same as RBI, $a$ impenetrant, $B'$ inviable

RBI, $A'$ impenetrant, $B'$ inviable
  Same as CBI, $a$ impenetrant, $b$ inviable

---

The single backcross produces to a total of 16 cases, depending upon the combination of the various parameters. The estimating formulae are presented in Table 7.6. Overall, these display a discernible pattern. The elements of the matrices which these cases generate are listed in Table 7.7. The pertinent variance is then:

$$V = \frac{D}{n(AD - B^2)}.$$

# CHAPTER 8

# Scoring

One of the attributes of estimation by maximum likelihood is the development of scores. These arise as part of the analytical procedure and can themselves lead to valid estimates of an unknown parameter or parameters. The explicit use of maximum likelihood scores was outlined by Fisher (1946). A more formalized approach was made by Finnery (1949), who also presented numerical tables of scores designed to facilitate the calculation of the crossover fraction. Allard (1956) has given tables of scores to cover a greater number of crosses. Scoring procedures have also been shortly considered by Kramer and Burham (1947), Mather (1951), Carter and Falconer (1951), Fisher and Yates (1953), Bailey (1961), and Green (1963).

The relative ease by which scores can be derived for the majority of crosses and the existence of tables of scores, has prompted the suggestion that estimation should be accomplished by the method alone. The method is certainly easy to apply and consultation of tables can reduce the amount of arithmetic. However, once an explicit estimating formula and variance has been derived for the various crosses, estimation by scoring has been effectively by-passed.

The calculation of a score is particularly useful for those cases where the estimating formula is an equation of cubic or higher degree. It is customary to solve equations of this type numerically and scoring is a convenient method. Several cases have been described in previous chapters, where such equations have been encountered. The initial value of $p$ which must be fitted into the score and variance can be chosen either by an intelligent guess or by an approximation derived from such parts of the data capable of yielding a simple estimator. The latter course has been recommended.

The routine adoption of scores should be used for the combination of segregations in the detection of weak linkages or to derive an estimate of the closest linkage consistent with apparently independent genes. The procedure is straightforward because numerical scores for most frequently recurring segregations can be listed for independent assortment and used repeatedly. This is equivalent to taking $p = 0.5$ and the $\chi^2$ test, which is derived from these scores, will be testing the segregation for deviation from independent assortment. Scoring and combining data in this manner is simulating a sequential analysis in essential features although possibly lacking the sophisticated approach of this technique (see McIntosh, 1956 and Andresen, 1968).

Table 8.1 lists scoring coefficients for $p = 0.5$ for many of the common segregations. The observed frequencies $a, b, \ldots$ represent the same phenotype class as defined in earlier sections. The numerical coefficients indicate the contribution of each class to the score $S$. The information, $I$, for each

TABLE 8.1

Scoring coefficients and information for testing independent assortment. Locus $a$ taken as epistatic recessive or dominant where applicable

| Cross | Score | Information per observation |
|---|---|---|
| RBB | $2a - 2b - 2c + 2d$ | 4 |
| RII | $\dfrac{4a}{9} - \dfrac{4b}{3} - \dfrac{4c}{3} + 4d$ | $\dfrac{16}{9}$ |
| RIB | $\dfrac{2a}{3} - \dfrac{2b}{3} - 2c + 2d$ | $\dfrac{4}{3}$ |
| RII, $B$ codominant | $\dfrac{4a}{3} - \dfrac{4c}{3} - d + f$ | $\dfrac{8}{3}$ |
| RII, $A$ and $B$ codominant | $4a - 4d$ | 4 |
| Rec. epistasis RBB | $2a - 2b$ | 4 |
| RII | $\dfrac{4a}{9} - \dfrac{4b}{3}$ | $\dfrac{16}{27}$ |

Table 8.1—*(Continued)*

| Cross | Score | Information per observation |
|-------|-------|---------------------------|
| RIB | $\dfrac{2a}{3} - \dfrac{2b}{3}$ | $\dfrac{4}{9}$ |
| RBI | $\dfrac{2a}{3} - 2b$ | $\dfrac{4}{3}$ |
| Dom. epistasis | | |
| RBB | $-2c + 2d$ | $4$ |
| RII | $-\dfrac{4c}{3} + 4d$ | $\dfrac{16}{3}$ |
| RIB | $-2c + 2d$ | $4$ |
| RBI | $-\dfrac{2c}{3} + 2d$ | $\dfrac{4}{3}$ |
| Rec. mimics | | |
| RBB | $2a - \dfrac{2b}{3}$ | $\dfrac{4}{3}$ |
| RII | $\dfrac{4a}{9} - \dfrac{4b}{7}$ | $\dfrac{16}{13}$ |
| Dom. mimics | | |
| RBB | $\dfrac{2a}{3} - 2b$ | $\dfrac{4}{3}$ |
| RII | $-\dfrac{4a}{15} + 4b$ | $\dfrac{16}{15}$ |
| $A'A'$ lethal | | |
| RII | $-\dfrac{4c}{3} + 4d$ | $\dfrac{16}{9}$ |
| RIB | $-2c + 2d$ | $4$ |
| RII, $B$ codominant | $-4c + 4d$ | $\dfrac{8}{3}$ |
| $A'A'$ and $B'B'$ lethal | | |
| RII | $-\dfrac{4a}{9} + \dfrac{8b}{9} + \dfrac{32c}{9}$ | $\dfrac{128}{81}$ |

Note: Rec. = recessive, Dom. = dominant, B = backcross, I = intercross for respective loci, R = repulsion. For coupling data, multiply all score coefficients by $-1$; the information is unchanged.

segregation is found by multiplying the information per single observation (right-hand column of the table) by the total number of observations, except in the case of epistasis and lethality. Where epistasis and lethality is involved, the information per single observation should be multiplied by the sum of the observations used to compute the score. The entries in the table are for repulsion phase; all of the scoring coefficients should be multiplied by $-1$ to convert these for use with coupling phase data. The information is unchanged.

Each segregation will yield a $\chi^2$ for one df as follows:

$$\chi^2 = \frac{S^2}{I},$$

where $S$ is the score and $I$ the amount of information at the value of the score. Each score has one df and summing the individual scores and information for $k$ segregations gives a total score with $k$ df:

$$\chi^2 = \frac{(\Sigma S)^2}{\Sigma I}$$

The individual $S$ may be either $+$ or $-$ and a check on possible between-segregation heterogeneity can be rapidly assessed by summing the $\chi^2$'s for the individual segregations and subtracting the total $\chi^2$ derived above. Symbolically, the calculation is:

$$\chi^2 = \Sigma \frac{S^2}{I} - \frac{(\Sigma S)^2}{\Sigma I}$$

and the difference has $k-1$ df.

Should the $\chi^2$ test be significant, linkage is indicated. The crossover fraction can be found by the explicit estimating formula for each segregation or by the continuation of the scoring. A provisional value can be found as:

$$p' = 0.5 + \frac{S}{I}$$

either for individual segregations or as a mean for the total. Note, $S$ will be negative for linkage. New scores are calculated for the provisional value $p'$ and the cycle of calculations is repeated. A second value of $p$ is found from the formula above.

If these data consist entirely or mostly of testcrosses, two cycles of calculation will usually suffice to reduce $S/I$ to a negligible value; otherwise, several cycles will probably be required.

Most of the algebraic expressions which are necessary for the scoring analysis are shown in Table 8.2. For convenience of presentation, the scores of the table are for repulsion phase. To convert these for coupling data, reverse the signs of each term (+ to $-$ and $-$ to +); and substitute $2(1-p)$ for $2p$ for all intercrosses. Similarly, substitute $(1-p)$ for $p$ in the formula for the information. Scores for intercrosses with codominant genes and homozygous lethals have been given in a previous chapter.

TABLE 8.2

Scoring coefficients and information for the more common repulsion phase crosses. Locus $a$ is taken as epistatic recessive or dominant where applicable. See text for details of conversion for use with coupling data

| Cross | Score | Information |
|-------|-------|-------------|
| RBB | $\dfrac{a}{p} - \dfrac{b}{1-p} - \dfrac{c}{1-p} + \dfrac{d}{p}$ | $\dfrac{1}{(1-p)p}$ |
| RII | $\dfrac{2ap}{2+p^2} - \dfrac{2bp}{1-p^2} - \dfrac{2cp}{1-p^2} + \dfrac{2dp}{p^2}$ | $\dfrac{2(1+2p^2)}{(2+p^2)(1-p^2)}$ |
| RIB | $\dfrac{a}{1+p} - \dfrac{b}{2-p} - \dfrac{c}{1-p} + \dfrac{d}{p}$ | $\dfrac{1+2(1-p)p}{2(1+p)(2-p)(1-p)p}$ |
| Rec. epistasis<br>RBB | $\dfrac{a}{p} - \dfrac{b}{1-p}$ | $\dfrac{1}{(1-p)p}$ |
| RII | $\dfrac{2ap}{2+p^2} - \dfrac{2bp}{1-p^2}$ | $\dfrac{4p^2}{(2+p^2)(1-p^2)}$ |
| RIB | $\dfrac{a}{1+p} - \dfrac{b}{2-p}$ | $\dfrac{1}{(1+p)(2-p)}$ |
| RBI | $\dfrac{a}{1+p} - \dfrac{b}{1-p}$ | $\dfrac{1}{(1+p)(1-p)}$ |
| Dom. epistasis<br>RBB | $-\dfrac{c}{1-p} + \dfrac{d}{p}$ | $\dfrac{1}{(1-p)p}$ |
| RII | $-\dfrac{2cp}{1-p^2} + \dfrac{2dp}{p^2}$ | $\dfrac{4}{1-p^2}$ |

Table 8.2—*(Continued)*

| Cross | Score | Information |
|---|---|---|
| RIB | $-\dfrac{c}{1-p}+\dfrac{d}{p}$ | $\dfrac{1}{(1-p)p}$ |
| RBI | $-\dfrac{c}{2-p}+\dfrac{d}{p}$ | $\dfrac{1}{(2-p)p}$ |
| Rec. mimics RBB | $\dfrac{a}{p}-\dfrac{b}{2-p}$ | $\dfrac{1}{p(2-p)}$ |
| RII | $\dfrac{a}{2+p^2}-\dfrac{b}{2-p^2}$ | $\dfrac{4p^2}{(2+p^2)(2-p^2)}$ |
| Dom. mimics RBB | $\dfrac{a}{1+p}-\dfrac{b}{1-p}$ | $\dfrac{1}{(1+p)(1-p)}$ |
| RII | $-\dfrac{a}{4-p^2}+\dfrac{b}{p^2}$ | $\dfrac{4}{4-p^2}$ |

Note: Rec. = recessive, Dom. = dominant, B = backcross, I = intercross for respective loci. R = repulsion.

When two genes are known to be linked, scoring may be employed to find the mean crossover value for a number of segregations although it is usually easier to do this by weighting with the respective amounts of information. Calculation of scores for a number of different types of segregations does, however, permit a simple analysis of between-segregation heterogeneity. Crossover values do vary between segregations for a number of reasons and it is useful to check for this. The ordinary $\chi^2$ tests for heterogeneity cannot be applied when it is desirable to compare, for example, testcrosses and intercrosses.

All segregations should be examined for normal gene ratios since none of the tabulated scores allow for disturbances due to inviability or impenetrance. When these are present, scores must be formulated which allow for these factors. The degree of inviability or impenetrance can be found by simultaneous estimation in conjunction with the crossover fraction. The inviability and impenetrance usually feature in the information and must, therefore, be estimated. This can be accomplished in most cases by explicit estimating formulae but should these be cubic or higher degree equations, simultaneous estimation is the practical method of tackling the problem. Chapter 2 outlines the general technique.

In calculating scores, it is often advisable to work throughout in terms of $p$, even for intercrosses. The means using $p^2$ or $(1-p)^2$ in place of $P$. However, if the latter is used, the score for $P$ can be converted to that for $p$, by employing the score multiplier listed in Table 2.3, according to the nature of the intercross.

# CHAPTER 9

# Multipoint Crosses

There have been few serious investigations of multi-point crosses among mammals, There are probably two reasons for this. In the first place, investigation of multi-point crosses requires an intensive level of analysis which has had few aspirants. In the second place, only fairly recently have extensive linked groups of genes become available which would make such analyses profitable. The way is now open for a more systematic study of multiple linkage, as opposed to opportunist use of such linked genes as are readily available. The analytical and statistical procedures have been thoroughly outlined in a number of publications (Owen, 1950, 1953b; Parsons, 1958; Bailey, 1961). A full and interesting discussion of many of the basic principles which should be followed has been provided by Wallace (1957a).

There are several items to emphasize in multi-point crosses. The most fundamental is that an effort should be made to obtain the maximum return for effort. Unless there are special reasons to the contrary, multiple testcrosses are preferable to single backcrosses or intercrosses. Genes with inviability or impenetrant effects should be avoided or, if this is impossible, not more than one gene with either of these complications should be included. The reason is that the subsequent statistical analysis would be needlessly complicated. Genes with epistatic effects should also be preferentially excluded because of the wastage due to incomplete classification. It is necessary to examine large samples, particularly if the linkages are small, to obtain adequate numbers of double crossover individuals and to reduce the standard errors of the coincidence and Kosambi coefficient to low values.

The most widely reported analysis has been the relatively simple three-point. Indeed, at the present stage of theory, there is little information to be obtained from the four-point and higher crosses which cannot be gained from the three-point. Once a gene has been assigned to a linkage group, a three-point cross is desirable. Although two-point crosses can locate a gene in the crossover map, the three-point can do this more efficiently. It can reduce the number of crosses at least by one and can usually provide a direct indication of the serial order of the genes. The median placed gene can only be separated from its fellows by double crossingover and the frequency of this class will be the lowest of those expected.

The three-point testcross can be analysed most expeditiously by a small rearrangement of the class expectations. The assorting offspring are classified phenotypically in the usual manner and the class frequencies should be examined for normal gene ratios. Then, instead of grouping the classes into non-recombinations and recombinations, these should be grouped as non-recombinations; recombination is the first segment (say, between loci $a$-$b$), recombination in the second segment (say, between loci $b$-$c$) and recombination in both segments (double recombinants). These four groups of classes are conventionally indicated by the symbols 0, 1, 2, and 12, respectively. Thus:

| Crossover types | 0 | 1 | 2 | 12 | Total |
|---|---|---|---|---|---|
| Observations | $a$ | $b$ | $c$ | $d$ | $n$ |

The crossover functions and variances follow immediately as:

| Gene pair | Crossover function | Variance |
|---|---|---|
| $a-b$ | $p_1 = \dfrac{b+d}{n}$ | $\dfrac{p_1(1-p_1)}{n}$ |
| $b-c$ | $p_2 = \dfrac{c+d}{n}$ | $\dfrac{p_2(1-p_2)}{n}$ |
| $a-c$ | $p_{1+2} = \dfrac{b+c}{n}$ | $\dfrac{p_{1+2}(1-p_{1+2})}{n}$ |

A fourth quantity, which will be required later, is:

$$z = \frac{d}{n}$$

and represents the rate of occurrence of double crossovers.

It will be seen that the sum of the two crossover functions for intercepts a-b and b-c will regularly exceed the crossover fraction for the a-c intercept because of the existence of double crossingover. In fact, if crossingover occurs at random, the three crossover fractions are connected as follows:

$$p_{1+2} = p_1 + p_2 - 2p_1 p_2.$$

The relation, however, only holds if either or both $p_1$ and $p_2$ are small. For moderate or large crossover fractions, observed values of $p_{1+2}$ differ from those expected and this has lead to the conceptions of interference. When crossingover occurs completely at random, $p_{12}$ should equal $p_1 p_2$. Usually, it does not and the ratio:

$$C = \frac{p_{12}}{p_1 p_2}.$$

has been defined as the coincidence. When $C$ is equal to unity, interference is nil and when less than unity, interference is present and positive. Negative interference is possible and would be indicated by a value greater than unity. These considerations have inspired the notion that the relation between $p_{1+2}$ and $p_1$ and $p_2$ could be more logically represented as:

$$p_{1+2} = p_1 + p_2 - 2C p_1 p_2,$$

by combining the above concepts.

At this point, it may seem desirable to estimate $C$ and this may be accomplished from two sets of data. Estimates of $p_1$, $p_2$, and $p_{1+2}$ may have been obtained from independent experiments, in which case, the estimator is:

$$C = \frac{p_1 + p_2 - p_{1+2}}{2p_1 p_2}$$

and

$$V = \frac{p_1^2 (p_{1+2} - p_1)^2 V_2 + p_2^2 (p_{1+2} - p_2)^2 V_1 + p_1^2 p_2^2 V_{1+2}}{4 p_1^4 p_2^4}$$

where $V_1$, $V_2$, and $V_{1+2}$ are the variances of $p_1$, $p_2$, and $p_{1+2}$, respectively, (Bailey, 1961). This estimator has been rarely utilized.

However, $C$ may be estimated more efficiently from the three-point cross. Assuming that the cross has been analysed for the various $p$'s and $z$, the estimator is (Stevens, 1936):

$$C = \frac{z}{p_1 p_2} = \frac{nd}{(b+d)(c+d)}$$

and

$$V = \frac{C[1 - C(p_1 + p_2) - p_1 p_2 C(1 - 2C)]}{n p_1 p_2}.$$

The coincidence has often been used in the older literature as an index of the degree of interference. The greater the deviation of $C$ from unity, the greater the interference. $C$ is satisfactory in this respect for assessing interference within a sample but less so as a measure of interference along the chromosome. In practice, $C$ has been found to be dependent on the length of the two intercepts involved, being lower for long intercepts (Owen, 1950; Wallace, 1957a). Partly to overcome this disadvantage, a somewhat more general index has been proposed and designated the Kosambi coefficient:

$$K = \frac{z}{2 p_1 p_2 p_{1+2}} = \frac{n^2 d}{2(b+c)(b+d)(c+d)}$$

and

$$V = \frac{K^2}{n} \left[ \frac{5}{p_{1+2}} + \frac{1}{z} + \frac{2z}{p_1 p_2} - \frac{1}{p_1} - \frac{1}{p_2} - 4 - 4K(p_1 + p_2) \right].$$

The interrelation between $K$ and $C$ is $K = C/2p_{1+2}$ (Owen, 1950, 1953b).

Owen (1950, 1953b) has deduced mathematically that $K$ will have a value greater than unity for regions of the chromosome near the centromere. The value decreases steadily for greater distances, becoming less than unity for the distal end of the arm. It is, therefore, conceivable that examination of $K$ values for triads of intercepts could give an indication of their position relative to the centromere. In particular, detection of a trend could locate the position of the centromere. If Owen's deductions are true, $K$ will approximately equal unity for the medial region of the chromosome. This is of practical interest since it implies that the Kosambi mapping function could hold for an important region of many chromosomes.

The significance of differences between $K$ values for various regions of the chromosome is presumably easily effected when the loci involved do not overlap. The difference may be treated as a normal deviate. The situation is more complicated when the loci overlap since the $K$'s are not then independent. Owen (1953b) has approached the situation when he considers four-point data. When the four loci (say, $a$, $b$, $c$, and $d$) are not sited so closely that double crossingover is infrequent, he recommends that the observations should be analysed as a pair of triads, viz., $a$-$b$-$c$ and $b$-$c$-$d$. The two estimates of $K$ may then be compared. The variance of the difference contains a covariance term and this is derived by Owen, but seemingly incorrectly according to Bailey (1961). Bailey's covariance expression contains 20 terms and the appropriate section (10.43) of this author's monograph should be consulted for full details.

The four-point cross with closely linked loci introduces the problem that double crossover individuals will be rare and the triple crossover class non-existent. Bailey (1953b) has derived an approximate formulae for $K$ which takes advantage of the fact that the sum of the three double crossover classes may be adequately represented. Let the observed frequencies of the various crossover classes be:

| Crossover types | 0 | 1 | 2 | 3 | 12 | 13 | 23 | 123 | Total |
|---|---|---|---|---|---|---|---|---|---|
| Observations | $a$ | $b$ | $c$ | $d$ | $e$ | $f$ | $g$ | 0 | $n$ |

The crossover fractions and variance are approximately:

| Gene pair | Crossover fraction | Variance |
|---|---|---|
| $a$-$b$ | $p_1 = \dfrac{b+e+f}{n}$ | $\dfrac{p_1(1-p_1)}{n}$ |
| $c$-$d$ | $p_2 = \dfrac{c+e+g}{n}$ | $\dfrac{p_2(1-p_2)}{n}$ |
| $d$-$e$ | $p_3 = \dfrac{d+f+g}{n}$ | $\dfrac{p_3(1-p_3)}{n}$ |

The approximate formulae for $K$ and variance are:

$$K = \frac{3sn^2}{2(s_1^3 - s_3)}$$

and

$$V = K^2 \left[ \frac{1}{s} + \frac{9(s_5 + s_1^5 - 2s_1^2 s_3)}{(s_1^3 - s_3)^2} - \frac{4}{n} \right],$$

where

$$s = e + f + g, \quad s_1 = b + c + d, \quad s_3 = b^3 + c^3 + d^3$$

$$\text{and} \quad s_5 = b^5 + c^5 + d^5.$$

The analysis of multi-point crosses attains its highest level of efficiency when it can be arranged for these to be fully and appropriately balanced. It is widely appreciated that balanced data for the two-point case means the examination of equal numbers of offspring from the two possible linkage phases (i.e. $++/ab$ and $+b/a+$). The same principle applies to higher point data. As the number of loci increases (which need not be linked as in the present context), so do the number of different heterozygous types and the minimum number of matings required to produce a balanced experiment (Fisher and Mather, 1936; Edwards, 1958). Table 9.1 shows the trend of these increases. Edwards discusses the logic of the situation and outlines a method of finding the minimum number of matings for successive numbers of loci.

Fisher and Mather give details of the composition of recommended sets of mating types for two to eight loci. For two and three loci, there is no choice of different sets. All of the heterozygous types have to be used in the experiment. For four loci, there is a choice between four different sets. That is, there is no need to use all of the eight different heterozygotes, only specific combinations. For more than four loci, the number of required mating types increases but nowhere quite so rapidly as the number of different heterozygotes. It is by no means certain that the same set of mating types will be satisfactory for all experiments. This is an item which requires further study. It could be an advantage for more precise planning of experiments or it could be a snare if ignored.

TABLE 9.1

Number of different heterozygotes and minimum number of mating types to produce a balanced multi-point cross

| No. of loci | 2 | 3 | 4 | 5 | 6 | 7 | 8 | 9 | 10 | 11 | 12 | 13 | 14 | 15 | 16 |
|---|---|---|---|---|---|---|---|---|---|---|---|---|---|---|---|
| Heterozygotes | 2 | 4 | 8 | 16 | 32 | 64 | 128 | 256 | 502 | 1004 | 2008 | 40016 | 80032 | 160064 | 320128 |
| Mating types | 2 | 4 | 4 | 8 | 8 | 8 | 8 | 12 | 12 | 12 | 12 | 16 | 16 | 16 | 16 |

When only one locus has an allele conferring inviability, the analysis can proceed in the usual manner, estimation being exactly as for two-point assortment. When two or more genes show inviability, the effects of the inviability should not, in general, be ignored. Several methods of allowing for the inviability have been proposed but the simpler and probably the more practical methods of Fisher (1949) and Parsons (1957a) are to be recommended (Bailey, 1961). Both Parsons and Bailey outline the procedures to be followed and give an illustrative example. The arithmetic is heavy but unavoidable under the circumstances. The fact that the experiment consists of balanced data is an advantage in this direction. It is of interest that in the data analysed by Parsons, the difference between the crossover values for the raw and corrected data was small, as if the balanced nature of the experiment had already introduced an essential degree of correction.

An alternative analysis treats the data in the style of a factorial experiment (Bodmer and Parsons, 1959a, b; Bodmer, 1959). The analysis now is more elaborate but more rewarding in that the expression of the inviability can be partitioned into main effects and various interactions. In general, the $n$-point cross is arranged as a $2^{n-1} \times 2^{n-1}$ Latin square and the variability broken down by analysis of variance. Bodmer and Parsons (1959a) discuss the three-point situation in some detail while their later paper (1959b) discusses four-point and higher point data. The use of minimum mating types for experiments with many genes could mean that it is impossible to analyse some interactions but this can be offset by the principle of confounding. Bodmer (1959) discusses the complications which could follow if the inviability effects are largely non-linear and proposes, in particular, that a logarithmic transformation of the data might be useful. Bailey (1961) has discussed some of the problems inherent in the factorial approach and especially the difficulties which may arise if the inviability effects are non-linear.

Impenetrance can be estimated reasonably simply for the two-point cross but less easily for the multi-point. A full maximum likelihood analysis has the appearance of being excessively complicated. An alternative procedure is to correct for the impenetrance by adjustment of the observed frequencies. This may result in some loss of efficiency and this aspect deserves examination. However, the corrective procedures are not difficult to apply and are described by Parsons (1957b) and Bailey (1961). The three-point situation is discussed in detail by both authors while Parsons indicates that the procedures can be readily extended to four-point and higher crosses. It is noteworthy that Parsons and Bailey give slightly different expressions for one of the variances. Parsons' method of arriving at these appear intuitively to be correct but Bailey considers that at least one of Parsons' derivations can be queried.

Some of the intricacies of maximum likelihood scoring of several simultaneously linked genes have been discussed by Rao (1950).

CHAPTER 10

# Mapping Functions

The raw data for chromosome mapping are the crossover values obtained for loci spaced serially along the physical chromosomes. The simplest map is that of the cumulative sum of crossover values for adjacent genes. This is the map expressed in crossover units. When the loci are sited close together, the cumulative sum gives an accurate representation of the chromosome in centimorgans. Unfortunately, when the loci are not sited close together, the simple one-to-one relationship breaks down. The greater distance, the poorer the representation. To bridge the gulf, it is necessary to derive a mapping function to relate the determined crossover value to chromosome segment length.

The reasons for non-linear relationship between crossover value and chromosome length are two: the occurrence of multiple crossingover and interference. Given a chromosome segment *a-b,* there is a definite probability that a second crossover will occur within it. However, as the segment increases in length, there is also the probability that a second crossover will occur. The two together will nullify each other. Hence, the crossover values will represent the probability that the total number of crossovers between the *a* and *b* loci will be odd. This is multiple crossingover and, if this was the only important factor, it would lead to a simple mapping function.

However, the distribution of crossingover points is not entirely at random. The occurrence of one crossover tends to inhibit the occurrence of another in its immediate neighbourhood. This is known as interference and arises from the behaviour and nature of chiasma upon the chromosomes. Following Mather (1938), chiasma may be visualized as a serial process, commencing from the centromere and recurring at intervals along the chromosome arm. The distance between each chiasma may vary although it seems that only two distances need be distinguished. The first is between the centromere and the first chiasma (the differential distance) which varies to some extent according to chromosome length. The second is between successive chiasmata after the first (interference distance) and appears to be relatively constant. Two types of chiasmata formation may be recognized in the comprehensive four-strand model. The occurrence of a second chiasma may or may not involve the same chromatid as the first. The forms are known as chiasma interference and chromatid interference, respectively, and are of interest for the particular reason that the latter may be responsible for the production of crossover values exceeding 50 crossover units (Owen, 1950; Carter and Robertson, 1952).

The fact that $p$ does not measure chromosome map length ($x$) is of considerable interest and has stimulated a number of highly theoretical studies. The problem is to devise a mapping function which can satisfactorily relate the crossover function to map length for most, if not all, values of $p$. The early studies were a mixture of intuitive reasoning and empirical curve fitting. Haldane (1919b), Kosambi (1944), and Carter and Falconer (1951) have each made useful contributions in this respect. Working from relatively simple concepts, the differential equation was derived:

$$\frac{\mathrm{d}p}{\mathrm{d}x} = 1 - (bp)^k.$$

$b$ and $k$ being constants. $b$ is usually taken as 2 to comply with the assumption that at $p = 0.5$, the rate of change has fallen to zero. $k$ governs the rate of approach to the limiting value of zero. The following values of $k$ produce the relationships:

| $k$ | $x$ |
|---|---|
| 1 | $-\frac{1}{2} \ln (1 - 2p)$ |
| 2 | $\frac{1}{2} \tanh^{-1} 2p$ |
| 4 | $\frac{1}{4}(\tanh^{-1} 2p + \tan^{-1} 2p)$. |

All of the formulae yield monotonically increasing values of $p$ for successive values of $x$. The first one was derived by

Haldane (1919b) and is sometimes featured in elementary discussions of mapping functions. It represents, in fact, the situation of multiple crossingover but no interference. In practice, however, the representation is not too accurate and the formula has been superseded by the second, which is due to Kosambi (1944). This relationship has proved to be a practical working formula for many purposes. This aspect has been enhanced by the availability of Table VII for the transformation of the correlation coefficient in Fisher and Yates (1953). By taking $r = 2p$ and $x = r/2$ conversion of $p$ to $x$ (or *vice versa*) is rapidly effected.

The third formula has been proposed by Carter and Falconer (1951) as providing a good fit to house mouse linkage data. Since the mouse is the most extensively investigated mammalian species, as regards linkage, this makes the formula worthy of attention. A conversion table is given later (Table 12.6) for use as an auxiliary tool in the analysis of mouse data. The Carter/Falconer function has emerged as superior to the Kosambi for the mouse and may indeed be generally superior for other mammalian species. The Kosambi and Carter/Falconer functions have been termed 'empirical' since their usefulness resides in ease of calculation and goodness of fit to observation rather than upon fundamental biological quantities.

Although the additive properties of the crossover value breaks down for loci which are not closely linked, a combination formula has been derived which is of remarkable utility. If $p_1$, $p_2$, and $p_{1+2}$ are the crossover fraction for the intercepts *a-b*, *b-c*, and *a-c*, respectively, then:

$$p_{1+2} = \frac{p_1 + p_2}{1 + 4p_1 p_2}.$$

This relation, although based on the Kosambi function, has been shown to hold good for a wide range of crossover values. It is apparently least accurate for weak linkages of about 30 or more crossover units and its use in this region should be viewed with caution. The existence of this formula is one reason for the popularity of the Kosambi mapping function. Unfortunately, it does not seem possible to extend the formula to more than three intercepts (but see Owen, 1953b for a discussion on how this disadvantage can be partially offset).

The development of a thoroughgoing theory of mapping functions, which is explicitly cognizant of the underlying biological variables, is a comparatively recent venture. In summary, these are the serial occurrence of chiasmata among the chromatid strands and their probability distributions as modified by the centromere and various forms of interference. The observations and concepts of Mather (1936b, 1937, 1938) on chiasma formation provided the basis for most of this work but not necessarily all. In a sense, this development had to wait until such concepts as Mather's had been advanced but, even so, there appears to have been a considerable time-lag. The reason seems to be that Kosambi's formula was adequate until Wright (1947) discovered significant linkage values in excess of 50 and that these were rather curiously interrelated. It was realized that the Kosambi relationship, while providing a creditable fit to observation, was not more than an inspired mathematical guess.

The first papers to deal with the problem are those of Fisher, Lyon, and Owen (1947) and Fisher (1948). These were followed by the detailed studies of Owen (1949, 1950, 1951), Carter and Robertson (1952), Payne (1956, 1957), Takashi (1957), and Walmsley (1969). Carter and Robertson objected to some aspects of Owen's analysis but Owen (1952, 1953a) showed that these objections are probably based on a misconception (Bailey, 1961). The fundamental contributions are those of Owen (1949, 1950) while prospective summaries are provided by Owen (1950) and Bailey (1961).

The analyses are highly mathematical and the original papers should be consulted for details. The most interesting findings are two. It is *a priori* probable that the derived functions will give a superior fit to observation for high crossover values and that, under certain conditions, crossover values in excess of 50 may be expected. This excess crossingover will only occur for a short segment of chromosome. For greater distances (measured from the centromere), the crossover value falls back to the 'random' value of 50 per cent recombination; or, alternatively, there is the possibility of damped oscillations for very long chromosome arms.

However, it is by no means certain that crossover values beyond 50 per cent will occur. For such values to exist, chromatid interference must be occurring above a certain minimum level and the chromosome arm will probably have to be fairly long (though this is variable according to the model; Carter and Robertson, 1952; Owen, 1953a). Carter and Robertson (1952) have considered the matter and reviewed the literature. The relevant data are either inconclusive or negative at that time. The early observations of Wright (1947) for the mouse have not been confirmed by independent experiments (Carter and Phillips, 1953; Tatchell, 1961a). The existence of excess crossover values depends primarily on a high level of chromatid interference and a specific investigation by Carter (1954) for the male mouse failed to detect such levels. If chromatid interference is present in this species, the level is low and may indeed be absent.

# General Bibliography

ALAM, M. (1929). The calculation of linkage values. *Mem. Dep. Agric. India, Bot. Ser.*, **18**, No. 1, 56 Pp.

ALLARD, R. W. (1956). Formulae and tables to facilitate the calculation of recombination values in heredity. *Hilgardia*, **24**, 235-278.

ALLARD, R. W. and ALDER, H. L. (1960). The effect of incomplete penetrance on the estimation of recombination values. *Heredity*, **15**, 263-282.

ANDRESEN, E. (1968). Sequential analysis of genetic linkage in pigs. *Roy. Vet. Agric. Coll. Copen. Yrb.* (1968), 1-11.

BAILEY, N. T. J. (1949a). The use of the product formula for the estimation of linkage when differential viability is present. *Heredity*, **3**, 220-225.

BAILEY, N. T. J. (1949b). A method for allowing for differential viability in estimating linkage from backcross matings in coupling only or repulsion only. *Heredity*, **3**, 225-228.

BAILEY, N. T. J. (1950). The influence of partial manifestation on the detection of linkage. *Heredity*, **4**, 327-336.

BAILEY, N. T. J. (1951). Testing the solubility of maximum likelihood equations in the routine application of scoring methods. *Biometrics*, **7**, 268-274.

BAILEY, N. T. J. (1961). *Introduction to the mathematical theory of genetic linkage.* London: Oxford University Press.

BHAT, N. R. (1950). Procedure for the measurement of linkage between characters determined by dissimilar factors with complete dominance. *Indian J. Genet. Plant Breed.*, **10**, 21-27.

BODMER, W. F. (1959). Multiplicative effects and the logarithmic transformation in the analysis of balanced multi-point linkage tests. *Heredity*, **13**, 157-164.

BODMER, W. F. and PARSONS, P. A. (1959a). The analogy between factorial experimentation and balanced multi-point linkage tests. *Heredity*, **13**, 145-156.

BODMER, W. F. and PARSONS, P. A. (1959b). Factorial analysis of balanced four and higher point linkage tests. *Heredity*, **13**, 157-164.

CARTER, T. C. (1951). The position of fidget in linkage group V of the house mouse. *J. Genet.*, **50**, 264-267.

CARTER, T. C. (1954). A search for chromatid interference in the male house mouse. *Z. Ind. Abst. Vererb.*, **86**, 210-223.

CARTER, T. C. (1957). The use of linked marker genes for detecting recessive autosomal lethals in the mouse. *J. Genet.*, **55**, 585-597.

CARTER, T. C. and FALCONER, D. S. (1951). Stocks for detecting linkage in the mouse and the theory of their design. *J. Genet.*, **50**, 307-323.

CARTER, T. C. and FALCONER, D. S. (1952). A review of independent segregation in the house mouse. *J. Genet.*, **50**, 399-413.

CARTER, T. C. and PHILLIPS, R. J. S. (1953). The sex distribution of waved-2, shaker-2 and rex in the house mouse. *J. Vererbungslehre*, **85**, 564-578.

CARTER, T. C. and ROBERTSON, A. (1952). A mathematical treatment of genetical recombination using a four strand model. *Proc. Roy. Soc.*, *B*, **139**, 410-426.

CASTLE, W. S. (1939). On a method of testing for linkage between lethal genes. *Proc. Nat. Acad. Sci, Wash.*, **25**, 593-594.

COCKRAN, W. G. (1954). Some methods for strengthening the common $\chi^2$ tests. *Biometrics*, **10**, 417-451.

COOPER, C. B. (1939). A linkage between naked and caracul in the house mouse. *J. Hered.*, **30**, 212.

DOUGLAS, L. T. and GEERTS, S. J. (1967). Meiosis II: a modified affinity model in mice. *Genetica*, **37**, 511-542.

EDWARDS, A. W. F. (1958). Number of mating types required for balance in multi-point linkage programmes. *Nature, Lond.*, **181**, 503-504.

FALCONER, D. S (1949). The estimation of mutation rates from incompletely tested gametes and the detection of mutations in mammals. *J. Genet.*, **49**, 226-234.

FINNERY, D. J. (1949). The estimation of the frequency of recombinants. I. Matings of known phase. *J. Genet.*, **49**, 159-176.

FISHER, R. A. (1922). On the mathematical foundations of theoretical statistics. *Phil. Trans. Roy. Soc.*, *A*, **122**, 309-368.

FISHER, R. A. (1939). The precision of the product formula for the estimation of linkage. *Ann. Eugen.*, **9**, 50-54.

FISHER, R. A. (1946). A system of scoring linkage data with special reference to pied factors in mice. *Amer. Nat.*, **80**, 568-578.

FISHER, R. A. (1948). A quantitative theory of genetic recombination and chiasma formation. *Biometrics*, **4**, 1-13.

FISHER, R. A. (1949). Note on the test of significance for differential viability in frequency data from a complete three point test. *Heredity*, **3**, 215-219.

FISHER, R. A (1951). *The design of experiments*. Edinburgh: Oliver and Boyd.

FISHER, R. A (1962). The detection of a sex difference in recombination values using double heterozygotes. *J. Theoret. Biol.*, **3**, 509-513.

FISHER, R. A. and BALMUKAND, B. (1928). The estimation of linkage from the offspring of selfed heterozygotes. *J. Genet.*, **20**, 79-92.

FISHER, R. A., LYON, M. F. and OWEN, A. R. G. (1947). The sex chromosome of the house mouse. *Heredity*, 1, 355-365.

FISHER, R. A. and MATHER, K. (1936). A linkage test with mice. *Ann. Eugen.*, 7, 265-280.

FISHER, R. A. and YATES, F. (1953). *Statistical tables for biological agricultural and medical research.* Edinburgh: Oliver and Boyd.

GREEN, M. C. (1963). Methods for testing linkage. In Burdette, W. J. (Editor) *Methodology in mammalian genetics.* San Francisco: Holden-Day.

HALDANE, J. B. S. (1919a). The probable errors of calculated linkage values and the most accurate method of determining gametic from certain zygotic series. *J. Genet.*, 8, 291-297.

HALDANE, J. B. S. (1919b). The combination of linkage values and the calculation of distance between the loci of linked factors. *J. Genet.*, 8, 299-309.

HALDANE, J. B. S. (1953). The estimation of two parameters from a sample. *Sankhya*, 12, 313-320.

HOLLANDER, W. F. (1953). The ABC's of genetics. *J. Hered.*, 44, 211-212.

HOLLANDER, W. F. (1955). Epistasis and hypostasis. *J. Hered.*, 46, 223-225.

HOLLANDER, W. F. (1964). Repulsive thoughts on coupling. *J. Hered.*, 55, 17-19.

HUTCHINSON, J. B. (1929). The application of the method of maximum likelihood to the estimation of linkage. *Genetics*, 14, 519-537.

IMMER, F. R. (1930). Formulae and tables for calculating linkage intensities. *Genetics*, 15, 81-89.

IMMER, F. R. (1931). The efficiency of the correlation coefficient for estimating linkage intensities. *Amer. Nat.*, 65, 567-572.

IMMER, F. R. (1934). Calculating linkage intensities from $F_3$ data. *Genetics*, 19, 119-136.

IMMER, F. R. and HENDERSON, M. T. (1943). Linkage studies in barley. *Genetics*, 28, 419-440.

KOSAMBI, D. D. (1944). The estimation of map distances from recombination values. *Ann. Eugen.*, 12, 172-175.

KRAMER, H. H. and BURHAM, C. R. (1947). Methods of combining linkage values from backcross, $F_2$ and $F_3$ genetic data. *Genetics*, 32, 379-390.

LUDWIG, W. (1934). Uber numerische Beziehungen der Crossingover-Werte untereinander. *Z. Ind. Abst. Ververb.*, 67, 58-95.

MATHER, K. (1935). The combination of data. *Ann. Eugen.*, 6, 399-410.

MATHER, K. (1936a). Types of linkage data and their value. *Ann. Eugen.*, 7, 251-264.

MATHER, K. (1936b). The determination of position in crossingover. I. *Drosophila melanogaster. J. Genet.*, 33, 207-235.

MATHER, K. (1937). The determination of position in crossingover. II. The chromosome length/chiasma frequency relation. *Cytologia, Fujii Jub. Vol.*, 514-526.

MATHER, K. (1938). Crossingover. *Biol. Rev.*, 13, 252-292.

MATHER, K. (1946). *Statistical analysis in biology.* London: Methuen.

MATHER, K. (1951). *The measurement of linkage in heredity.* London: Methuen.

MCINTOSH, W. B. (1956). Linkage in *Peromyscus* and sequential tests for independent assortment. *Contr. Lab. Vert. Biol. Univ. Mich.,* 73, 1-27.

MICHIE, D. (1953). Affinity: a new genetic phenomenon in the house mouse. Evidence from distant crosses. *Nature, Lond.,* 171, 26-27.

MITCHIE, D. (1955). Affinity. *Proc. Roy. Soc. B.,* 144, 241-259.

MURTY, V. N. (1954a). The calculation of linkage values by Fisher's scoring method. *Indian J. Genet. Plant. Breed.,* 14, 39-43.

MURTY, V. N. (1954b). Estimation of linkage by the method of minimum discrepancy. *Genetics,* 39, 581-586.

OWEN, A. R. G. (1949). The theory of genetical recombination. I. Long chromosome arms. *Proc. Roy. Soc. B.,* 136, 67-94.

OWEN, A. R. G. (1950). The theory of genetical recombination. *Advanc. Genet.,* 3, 117-157.

OWEN, A. R. G. (1951). An extension of Kosambi's formula. *Nature, Lond.,* 168, 208.

OWEN, A. R. G. (1952). Four-strand crossingover. *Nature, Lond.,* 170, 985.

OWEN, A. R. G. (1953a). Super-recombination in the sex chromosome of the mouse. *Heredity,* 7, 103-110.

OWEN, A. R. G. (1953b). The analysis of multiple linkage data. *Heredity,* 7, 247-264.

PARSONS, P. A. (1957a). An effect of gene arrangement on the recombination fraction in *Drosophila melanogaster. Heredity,* 11, 117-127.

PARSONS, P. A. (1957b). Partial manifestation of a gene in complete three and higher point backcross data. *Heredity,* 11, 217-222.

PARSONS, P. A. (1958). A survey of genetic interference in maize. *Genetica,* 29, 222-237.

RAO, C. R. (1948). Large sample tests of statistical hypothesis concerning several parameters with applications to problems of estimation. *Proc. Camb. Phil. Soc.,* 44, 50-57.

RAO, C. R. (1950). Methods of scoring linkage data giving the simultaneous segregation of three factors. *Heredity,* 4, 37-59.

RAO, C. R. (1952). *Advanced statistical methods in biometrical research.* London: Chapman and Hall.

RIEGER, R., MICHAELIS, A. and GREEN, M. M. (1968). *A glossary of genetics and cytogenetics.* Berlin: Springer Verlag.

SANCHEZ-MONGE, E. (1952). The estimation of linkage with incomplete penetrance. *Heredity,* 6, 121-125.

SEAL, K. C. (1957). Generalization of product formula. *J. India Soc. Agric. Statist.,* 9, 31-40.

SHULT, E. E., DESBOROUGH, S. and LINDEGREN, C. C. (1962). Preferential segregation in *Saccharomyces. Genet. Res.,* 3, 196-209.

SCHULT, E. E., LINDEGREN, G. and LINDEGREN, C. C. (1967). Hybrid specific linkage relations in *Saccharomyces. Canad. J. Genet. Cytol.*, **9**, 723-759.

SRINATH, K. V. (1949). The mechanics of crossingover. *Proc. Roy. Soc. B.*, **136**, 126-130.

STEVENS, W. L. (1936). The analysis of interference. *J. Genet.*, **32**, 51-64.

STEVENS, W. L. (1939). Tables of the recombination fraction estimated from the product ratio. *J. Genet.*, **39**, 171-180.

STEVENS, W. L. (1942). Accuracy of mutation rates. *J. Genet.*, **43**, 301-307.

TAKASHI, I. (1957). The theory of crossingover. *Jap. J. Genet.*, **32**, 189-193.

WALLACE, M. E. (1953). Affinity: a new genetic phenomenon in the house mouse. Evidence from within laboratory stocks. *Nature, Lond.*, **171**, 27-28.

WALLACE, M. E. (1957a). A balanced three-point experiment for linkage group V of the house mouse. *Heredity*, **11**, 223-258.

WALLACE, M. E. (1957b). The use of affinity in chromosome mapping. *Biometrics*, **13**, 98-110.

WALLACE, M. E. (1958). Experimental evidence for a new genetic phenomenon. *Phil. Trans. Roy. Soc., B.*, **241**, 211-254.

WALLACE, M. E. (1959). An experimental test of the hypothesis of affinity. *Genetica*, **29**, 243-255.

WALLACE, M. E. (1961). Affinity: evidence from crossing inbred lines of mice. *Heredity*, **16**, 1-23.

WALMSLEY, R. H. (1969). The general theory of mapping functions for random genetic recombination. *Biophys. J.*, **9**, 421-431.

WRIGHT, M. E. (1947). Two sex-linkages in the house mouse with unusual recombination values. *Heredity*, **1**, 349-354.

# Index to Part A

149

The index for Part B together with a consolidated index for both parts will appear at the end of Part B.